T0122826

Autonomous Unmanned Aerial Vehicles for Blood Delivery

A UAV Fleet Design Tool and Case Study

CHRISTOPHER K. GILMORE, MICHAEL CHAYKOWSKY, BRENT THOMAS

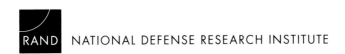

NATIONAL DEFENSE RESEARCH INSTITUTE

Prepared for the Office of the Secretary of Defense
Approved for public release

For more information on this publication, visit www.rand.org/t/RR3047

Library of Congress Cataloging-in-Publication Data is available for this publication.
ISBN: 978-1-9774-0346-9

Published by the RAND Corporation, Santa Monica, Calif.
© Copyright 2019 RAND Corporation
RAND® is a registered trademark.

Cover: U.S. Army/SFC Michael Guillory.

Support RAND
Make a tax-deductible charitable contribution at
www.rand.org/giving/contribute

www.rand.org

Preface

Autonomous unmanned aerial vehicles (UAVs) are becoming increasingly popular and have many potential applications. This analysis considers autonomous UAVs for medical resupply missions, in particular a blood delivery case study. We develop a design optimization tool that allows users to quickly assess small UAV designs. We believe the framework offered in this report will be most useful to acquisition program officials and Joint medical community stakeholders in understanding the requirements, capabilities, and cost drivers of small UAV delivery systems. Our approach is also readily applicable to other mission types.

This research was sponsored by the Office of the Secretary of Defense and conducted within the Acquisition and Technology Policy Center of the RAND National Defense Research Institute (NDRI), a federally funded research and development center (FFRDC) sponsored by the Office of the Secretary of Defense, the Joint Staff, the Unified Combatant Commands, the Navy, the Marine Corps, the defense agencies, and the defense Intelligence Community. For more information on the Acquisition and Technology Policy Center, see www.rand.org/nsrd/ndri/centers/atp or contact the director (contact information is provided on the webpage).

Contents

Figures

Tables

Summary

Autonomous unmanned aerial vehicles (UAVs) are quickly proliferating in both commercial and military markets. In the coming decade, the number of potential applications is also expected to expand. These applications include environmental monitoring, autonomous delivery, data collection, and photography and video. The advantages of these systems are certainly attractive—they minimize risk to operators, provide on-demand capability, and allow increased flexibility for reaching denied areas. In particular, the Joint medical community is interested in how autonomous UAVs can provide improved medical care capability, including medical resupply and unmanned casualty evacuation.

Despite their interest, the Joint medical community currently lacks a framework to assess the potential utility of autonomous UAVs for their missions. As such, this analysis aims to provide this analytic framework. We specifically focus on autonomous UAVs for blood delivery, a subset of the medical resupply mission space, for both logistical resupply of medical treatment facilities (MTFs) and emergency delivery to traumatically injured forward operators. Blood makes for an interesting UAV delivery case study because it has unique constraints regarding how it must be transported and stored and also has a finite shelf life. In short, blood could potentially benefit from a pairing with a delivery platform that allows for greater flexibility in its supply chain.

This analysis has three primary objectives: (1) Determine the required capability of a blood delivery UAV and define the corresponding mission space; (2) generate a UAV design that delivers this capability; and (3) understand the mission parameters that drive this design. To meet these objectives, we begin by first conducting a literature review and engaging Joint medical community stakeholders to define a notional blood delivery mission space (i.e., distances, payloads, and response times). With the mission space defined, we then develop a tool that optimizes small UAV designs based on a user-defined objective. The tool, which we call the Rapid UAV Design Optimization of Fixed-Wing Fleets (RUDOFF), generates globally optimal designs very quickly, making it ideal for conceptual design analyses and understanding high-level trade-offs that may be relevant to Joint medical stakeholders and acquisition program officials. We use RUDOFF to generate designs of blood delivery UAVs and to understand their most important design and cost drivers.

Table S.1 summarizes the notional mission space derived from a combination of literature review and stakeholder engagement. In particular, UAVs would ideally perform emergency deliveries within approximately 15 minutes, as transfusions for resuscitative care can improve survival outcomes if initiated within this time. Our literature review also yielded additional insights: (1) Several military research programs could make use of flexible and quickly composable logistical platforms—for example, autonomous medical resupply UAVs could quickly redistribute blood in response to a mass-casualty event; (2) recent UAV blood delivery flight tests have shown limited impact on blood quality, implying delivery via UAV would not adversely affect quality of care; and (3) onboard temperature control systems, if necessary during flight and post-delivery, should seek to maintain blood temperatures between 1°C and 6°C, the common standard for storage, not transport, of liquid blood products.

Table S.1
Notional Mission Space of a Blood Delivery, Autonomous UAV for Logistical Resupply and Emergency Delivery

Parameter	Logistical Resupply	Emergency Delivery
Range	~100 miles	~10 miles
Time	1 hour	15 minutes
Payload	10+ blood units	1 to 3 units

Using the notional mission space from Table S.1, we then use RUDOFF to estimate the optimal small blood delivery UAV design. We define the objective function that the tool seeks to minimize as the estimated life-cycle cost of the platform. This cost includes development, procurement, and sustainment costs for an assumed fleet size and system lifetime. We perform this analysis for two cases: (1) a single platform that flies both logistical and emergency missions and (2) two separate platforms that are mission-specific. Based on our definition of the UAV life-cycle cost, we find the single-platform solution to be the most cost-effective—that is, the cost of developing a second, additional platform outweighs the benefits of having two UAVs specifically tailored to each mission type. We note, however, that alternative definitions of the objective functions can potentially lead to different conclusions regarding fleet composition; for certain objective function definitions, the two mission-specific UAVs may be the optimal choice.

As the single platform performs both the logistical and emergency missions, we refer to this design as the one-size-fits-all solution. Figure S.1 provides an illustration of this optimal configuration. Table S.2 provides context for our design and compares the dimensions and weight of the one-size-fits-all UAV to the AeroVironment RQ-11B, a military reconnaissance small UAV platform, and the Zipline Zip 1, a commercial blood delivery autonomous aircraft. We find that our platform is both larger and heavier than the existing military option and has more demanding payload requirements than the existing commercial platform.

RUDOFF also generates UAV design sensitivities—in this case, these quantities represent the percent change in cost given a percent change in mission or design parameter, as noted in the bottom panel of Figure S.1. We see that this one-size-fits-all platform is most sensitive to the range requirement for the logistical resupply mission—that is, a 50-percent increase in the range constraint would increase total life-cycle costs by 70 percent. We also see that cost is less sensitive to the specified response times such that higher-speed UAVs would not cost as much as longer-range or larger-payload aircraft. We believe the framework offered in this analysis will be most useful to acquisition program officials and Joint medical community stakeholders who need

Figure S.1
Illustration of Optimal Design and Cost Sensitivities (Percent Change in Life-Cycle Cost for a 1-Percent Change in Mission Parameter) for the One-Size-Fits-All UAV

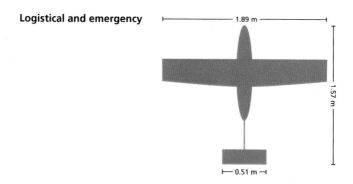

Logistical and emergency

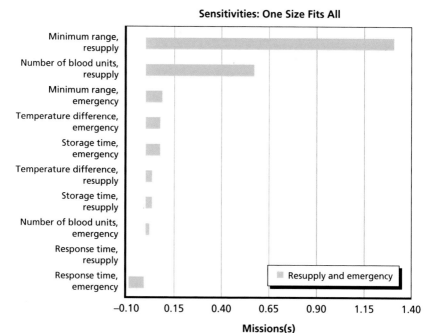

Sensitivities: One Size Fits All

Missions(s)
% change in cost for a 1% change in mission parameter

Table S.2
Design Specifications of the AeroVironment RQ-11B Raven, Zipline Zip 1, and Our One-Size-Fits-All Platform

Platform	Wingspan (m)	Chord (m)	Weight (kg)	Payload (kg)
RQ-11B Raven	1.37	0.22	1.9	0.2
Zip 1	1.83	0.24	12–14	1.5[a]
One-Size-Fits-All	1.89	0.33	39.9	10

SOURCES: AeroVironment, 2017a; RUDOFF tool; Stewart, 2017.
[a] Authors' estimate.

to understand the requirements, capabilities, and cost drivers of small UAV delivery systems.

Finally, we consider this analysis an initial assessment of a single medical resupply application that sits within a much larger mission space. Future RAND studies could use RUDOFF to assess other medical resupply missions, including assessing a single platform that serves a variety of purposes beyond the two assumed in this analysis. RUDOFF can also be more broadly applied to other mission types (e.g., intelligence gathering, reconnaissance). Stakeholders and researchers can generate similar information for any application as presented in this report.

Acknowledgments

There are a number of people in the Joint medical community that deserve credit for motivating and informing this work. We would like to thank LTC Ethan Miles from the 75th Ranger Regiment HQ for his help in starting RAND's work in blood logistics. Special thanks also go to COL Andrew Cap of the Army Institute of Surgical Research for his invaluable insight. We would also like to thank LCDR Steven Clifford and LTC Chris Evans of the U.S. Pacific Command (PACOM) and European Command (EUCOM) blood program offices; LTC Jessica Hughes, LTC Jason Corley, and CDR Jonathan Hoiles from the Armed Services Blood Program; and Dr. Gary Gilbert from Army MEDCOM for their help and motivating presence in this space.

At RAND, we would like to thank Christopher Mouton, Laura Baldwin, and Joel Predd for electing to fund and support this Office of the Secretary of Defense–sponsored research effort. Thanks also to Megan Mckeever for her help in project management. Finally, we thank the reviewers, Jia Xu, Bryan Boling, and Tony DeCicco, for their very helpful insights for improving this document.

Abbreviations

AABB	American Association of Blood Banks
AACUS	Autonomous Aerial Cargo/Utility System
ACES	Aircraft Concept Exploration System
AGL	above ground level
CER	cost-estimating relationship
DoD	Department of Defense
FAA	Federal Aviation Administration
FOF	fleet objective function
GA	genetic algorithm
GP	geometric programming
ISR	intelligence, surveillance, and reconnaissance
JMPT	Joint Medical Planning Tool
MGTOW	maximum gross takeoff weight
MTF	medical treatment facility
NACA	National Advisory Committee for Aeronautics
RBCs	red blood cells
RDT&E	research, development, test, and evaluation
RUDOFF	Rapid UAV Design Optimization of Fixed-wing Fleets
UAV	unmanned aerial vehicle
VTOL	vertical takeoff and landing

CHAPTER ONE

Introduction

Use of unmanned aerial vehicles (UAVs) is predicted to grow in the coming years across a number of sectors. Commercial sales, for example, are projected to grow 36 percent annually between 2018 and 2022 because of a growing number of potential applications, including environmental monitoring, aerial photography, and data collection (Business Wire, 2018b). The military UAV market is also expected to continue its historical growth at 4 percent per year between 2018 and 2028, driven primarily by demand for unmanned combat aerial vehicles and long-endurance platforms (Business Wire, 2018a).

UAVs vary widely in size and capability and fly different sets of missions. To distinguish between platforms, the Department of Defense (DoD) classifies its systems into "groups" defined by maximum gross takeoff weight (MGTOW), operating altitude, and airspeed, as reproduced in Table 1.1. As can be seen, military systems cover a wide spectrum, from the lighter, lower-flying, and slower Group 1 platforms, such as the RQ-11B Raven, to the heavier but longer-range and larger-payload Group 5 platforms, such as the MQ-9 Reaper (U.S. Air Force, 2019). These example platforms are shown in Figure 1.1. Separately, the Federal Aviation Administration (FAA) specifically distinguishes the "small" UAV as any platform that weighs less than 55 pounds, operates below 400 feet, and flies slower than 100 miles per hour (FAA, 2018)—that is, a Group 1 or 2 system. The term *micro-UAV* has also recently become more popular with the advent of UAV "swarm" concepts, referring to small geomet-

Table 1.1
DoD UAV Group Classifications with Examples

Group	MGTOW	Operating Altitude	Airspeed	Example
1	<20 lbs	<1,200 ft AGL	<100 knots	RQ-11B Raven
2	<55 lbs	<3,500 ft AGL	<250 knots	ScanEagle
3	<1,320 lbs	<18,000 ft MSL	<250 knots	RQ-7B Shadow
4	>1,320 lbs	<18,000 ft MSL	Any	MQ-1 Predator
5	>1,320 lbs	>18,000 ft MSL	Any	MQ-9 Reaper

SOURCE: U.S. Army, 2010.
NOTES: AGL = above ground level; MSL = mean sea level.

ric and aerodynamic scales on the order of tens of centimeters or less, of the corresponding platforms.[1]

More recently, commercial firms and the military have both recognized the potential of UAVs in autonomous delivery applications. Recent RAND work assessed the utility, deployment, and potential regulatory challenges of autonomous delivery drone fleets (Kuhn, 2017; Lohn, 2017; Xu, 2017).[2] Companies are also actively pursuing platforms, both large and small, for a variety of resupply missions.[3] Not surprisingly, autonomous delivery has drawn considerable interest from the military—unmanned systems minimize risk to personnel and the autonomy offers a flexible capability in the face of chaotic or uncertain operating environments. Recent DARPA initiatives, such as

---

[1]   The Air Force's micro-UAV Perdix, for example, highlights the limitation of the group classifications, as it does not neatly fall into any of these categories, given its relatively slow speed but high-altitude mission envelope. See Tao and Hansman (2016) for a more detailed description of the Perdix.

[2]   Note that this set of RAND studies used the term "drones," which is sometimes also interchangeably used with UAV. Popular usage, however, typically associates drones with quadcopters (e.g., the DJI Phantom), which are not the focus of this study.

[3]   See, for example, Elroy Air's autonomous UAV, which has been designed for commercial cargo, disaster relief, and military resupply missions (Elroy Air, undated).

Figure 1.1
The Group 1 RQ-11B Raven (Top) and the Group 5 MQ-9 Reaper (Bottom)

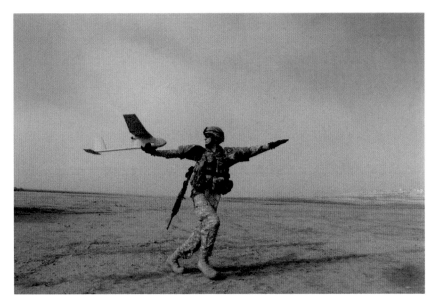

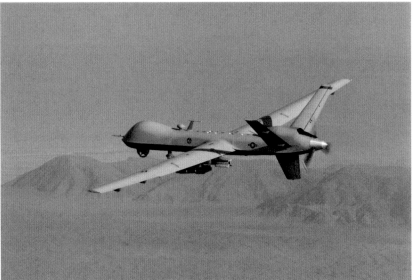

SOURCES: U.S. Army/SFC Michael Guillory (top); U.S. Air Force Photo / Lt. Col. Leslie Pratt (bottom).

CASCADE,[4] CONCERTO,[5] SoSITE,[6] and Mosaic,[7] also emphasize the benefit of rapidly composing mission capability from a large pool of low-cost assets, with autonomous systems partly enabling those visions. In addition, there are several ongoing military autonomous resupply research and development programs. One example is the Office of Naval Research's Autonomous Aerial Cargo/Utility System (AACUS) effort that is developing an on-demand, autonomous delivery helicopter. AACUS, developed by Aurora Flight Sciences, recently conducted its first operational test flight (Kucinski, 2018).

The Joint medical community, more specifically, is greatly interested in the utility offered by autonomous, unmanned systems. UAVs could be useful for medical resupply, both in military and civilian applications.[8] With regard to the military, autonomous UAVs could be used to quickly deliver emergency supplies on-demand during combat operations, such as in support of medical response to a mass-casualty event. With regard to civilian use, supplies could be flown into difficult-to-reach locations that may have been denied by a natural disaster or other catastrophic event. A more recent RAND study conducted by Thomas et al. (2018) specifically proposed the use of UAVs for alleviating logistical challenges within the Joint medical community's blood product supply chain.

---

[4]   The Complex Adaptive System Composition and Design Environment (CASCADE) program seeks to "fundamentally change how systems are designed for real-time resilient response to dynamic, unexpected contingencies." See Paschkewitz (2019) for a description of CASCADE.

[5]   See Javorsek (2019) for a description of CONverged Collaborative Elements for RF Task Operations (CONCERTO).

[6]   See Jones (2019) for a description of System of Systems Integration Technology and Experimentation (SoSITE).

[7]   The Defense Advanced Research Projects Agency (DARPA) "mosaic warfare" concept aims to bring together inexpensive systems to "enable diverse, agile applications." These systems are intended to be rapidly "tailored to accommodate available resources, adapt to dynamic threats, and be resilient to losses and attrition." See DARPA (2017).

[8]   The Joint medical community has also expressed interest in autonomous unmanned casualty evacuation platforms, although this is not without ethical concerns. This analysis only considers the medical resupply space, although future assessments could consider casualty evacuation.

Blood products, such as whole blood, plasma, red blood cells (RBCs), and platelets, make for an interesting UAV delivery case study.[9] Blood has unique constraints regarding how it must be transported and stored, and it has a finite shelf life—in short, blood could potentially benefit from a pairing with a delivery platform that could allow greater flexibility in its supply chain. For example, these supplies could be collected, stored, and used all in different locations with less impact on immediate availability. In addition, the mission space is potentially multidimensional: A UAV could be tasked to resupply a medical treatment facility (MTF) capable of properly storing blood, or perhaps that UAV could conduct emergency deliveries to forward operators to begin combat casualty resuscitative care as soon as possible.

In the civilian blood delivery space, Zipline has been one of the more successful ventures. Currently operating in Rwanda with plans to expand into nearby countries, Zipline has recently deployed the second version of its autonomous blood delivery fixed-wing[10] UAV, the Zip 2, shown in Figure 1.2. This more advanced platform is capable of delivering a 3.85-pound payload (i.e., sufficient for at least one unit of whole blood) at speeds nearing 80 miles per hour (Petrova and Koldony, 2018). Most important, however, Rwandan hospitals have made real use of these systems, allowing for blood storage centers to quickly distribute units to more remote medical facilities, bypassing slower and less reliable transportation infrastructure.

Motivation and Methods

Given the success of Zipline and the potential benefit to the Joint medical community, this analysis assesses autonomous delivery of blood

---

[9] With the exception of specifically referenced blood components and other products made from whole blood, we will, from this point forward, refer to blood and blood products more simply as *blood*.

[10] Fixed-wing is the conventional configuration of aircraft (e.g., commercial jets) and is distinct from tilt rotor or vertical takeoff and landing (VTOL) aircraft whose operation is similar to a helicopter.

Figure 1.2
The Zipline Zip 2 Fixed-Wing UAV for Blood Delivery Missions in Rwanda

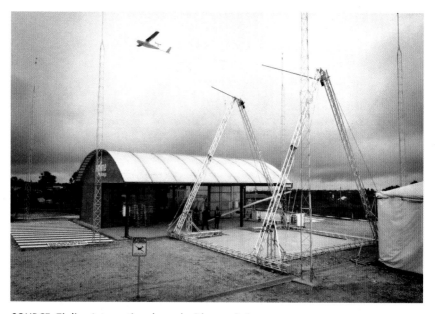

SOURCE: Zipline International, used with permission.

by small,[11] fixed-wing UAVs.[12] In particular, we envision two possible operational concepts:

- For logistical resupply of MTFs, UAVs are flown continuously or on-demand from a central blood storage facility to more remote MTFs that lack organic refrigeration capability. Each UAV has sufficient payload capacity to resupply a significant fraction of the MTF stores (i.e., on the order of 10 units).

---

[11] We use the term *small* flexibly in this report. While the FAA definition sets a weight limit, we use this classification to mean that the size of the UAV is on the order of a few meters.

[12] When we think of flight vehicles in the delivery context, existing proposed platforms (e.g., Google Wing and Amazon Prime Air) naturally conjure images of small-scale UAV systems with dimensions similar to the average human. This is not by accident, as the proposed payloads and delivery ranges subsequently demand aircraft of this size. As will be seen in Chapter Four, the UAV design we ultimately generate is of this scale.

- For emergency delivery to critically injured forward operators, UAVs are kept at forward MTFs or rerouted from other logistical functions and dispatched on-demand. Each vehicle carries enough blood for transfusion to one or two individuals (i.e., on the order of three units) and flies at sufficiently high speed to improve the survival outcome of the injured person. The design of this UAV is likely more sensitive to the trade-off between higher-speed and larger-payload deliveries.

In both cases, the UAV offloads its payload via airdrop and then makes its return journey, having sufficient fuel for both the outbound and inbound legs. In addition, multiple UAVs from the same or different locations could be dispatched to a single location if multiple logistical resupplies or emergency deliveries are required and a single vehicle payload is not sufficient.

Discussions with RAND subject matter experts make clear that the Joint medical community, despite having interest, lacks a framework in which to assess potential options to provide this capability, including what kind of flight vehicle they require and what mission parameters drive the design of such a UAV. As such, this analysis has three primary objectives: (1) Determine the required capability of a blood delivery UAV and define the corresponding mission space; (2) generate a UAV design that delivers this capability; and (3) understand the mission parameters that drive this design. Ultimately, we hope to provide relevant information that is useful to Joint medical stakeholders and acquisition program officials when developing and setting the requirements for a small UAV program.

To meet these objectives, we begin by first conducting a literature review of relevant topics that further motivate the utility of a blood delivery UAV—that is, how they can help mitigate logistical challenges and why faster delivery of blood for forward resuscitative care can lead to better survival outcomes. We also consider issues specific to transporting blood by small UAV, such as the relevant storage standards and whether the associated accelerations and environmental conditions can significantly degrade blood quality. Finally, with the help of Joint medical community subject matter experts, we define a notional blood delivery mission space (i.e., distances, payloads, and necessary delivery times) used later in the analysis to design a prospective UAV platform.

With the mission space defined, we then develop a design tool that is able to optimize the UAV based on a user-defined objective function. The tool, which we call the Rapid UAV Design Optimization of Fixed-Wing Fleets (RUDOFF), generates optimal small UAV designs very quickly by exploiting the convexity of the design problem, discussed in more detail in Chapter Three. This makes RUDOFF ideal for conceptual design analyses and understanding high-level trade-offs that may be relevant to stakeholders or acquisition program officials. For a given solution, RUDOFF also outputs design sensitivities to the defined objective function, allowing users to understand the most important drivers of the UAV design. For example, if an analyst defines the objective function to be the total life-cycle cost of the UAV, as we do in Chapter Four, then the design sensitivities correspond to the most important cost drivers. Finally, RUDOFF also offers the capability to define multiple UAV platforms and solve the corresponding mission assignment problem. This allows users to determine if single or multiple UAV types best span the mission space. In summary, this tool provides a systematic framework to conduct aircraft conceptual design analysis and understand the primary design trade-offs relevant for developing small UAV acquisition programs.

Outline

The remainder of this report is organized as follows: Chapter Two considers the technical details of transporting blood onboard small UAVs. It concludes by defining a notional blood delivery mission space to be applied in the remainder of the analysis. Chapter Three describes RUDOFF, the small UAV design optimization tool developed for this effort and includes a high-level overview of the model architecture and select model components. Chapter Four applies RUDOFF to design and assess a blood delivery UAV for both logistical resupply and emergency delivery missions. This assessment also provides cost sensitivities that allow stakeholders to understand how additional platform capability translates to additional program costs. Finally, Chapter Five concludes this report and offers a discussion of potential future applications and tool improvements.

CHAPTER TWO

Defining the Blood Delivery Mission Space

The mission space ultimately drives the design of any aircraft. This chapter describes how we define the blood delivery mission space and characterize potential constraints. We begin with a discussion of blood transport logistics and standards. We then consider the movement of blood specifically by small UAV and discuss related advantages and potential challenges. Next, we motivate the use of small UAVs for emergency blood delivery to forward locations, given potential improvements in survival outcomes for injured personnel. Then, we briefly discuss how operations within a contested environment might constrain the operation of delivery platforms. Finally, we conclude by summarizing the mission space used to generate optimal UAV designs in Chapter Four.

For a more in-depth analysis and assessment of the current Joint blood network, we refer readers to Thomas et al. (2018).

Logistical Advantages of Autonomous Delivery

As summarized in Thomas et al. (2018), the military's blood supply-chain network is both large in spatial extent and complex in its design. Blood requires careful testing, careful handling during transport, and storage, often with consistent temperature management. Moreover, system logistics are further complicated by the limited shelf lives of blood and blood products. Figure 2.1 provides a simplified illustration of the blood logistics network that highlights sources and sinks struc-

Figure 2.1
A Qualitative Framework of Blood Supply-Chain Flows and Processes

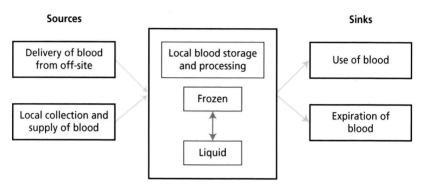

SOURCE: Adapted from Thomas et al., 2018.

tured around the storage of both frozen and liquid products.[1] These products typically come in four varieties: whole blood (i.e., blood collected directly from donors) and the components that can be readily separated from whole blood—namely, red blood cells (RBCs), plasma, and platelets. Transfusions can include any or all of these products, where RBCs, plasma, and platelets can be combined in some ratio to approximate whole blood. Thomas et al. (2018) also highlight how fragile the blood supply chain could be in a future large-scale conflict. Such an event, for example, could stress the network with a large number of trauma casualties in need of blood, coupled with degraded access to transportation for resupply of blood at forward-operating locations.

Given this issue, the Joint medical community has expressed interest in using autonomous UAVs to offer one flexible option to mitigate issues caused by supply-chain stressors. The specific advantages of autonomous systems are briefly summarized later in this chapter, but this potential capability is compelling for two reasons. First, autonomous UAVs offer a way to directly connect more remote blood collection or storage locations to MTFs. Second, such platforms could also

---

[1]   Frozen product shelf lives are typically longer than their liquid counterparts.

offer a means to quickly redistribute blood in theater in the event of some spike in local demand. Both of these advantages could make the blood supply network more resilient in future conflicts. The remainder of this section discusses the standards for blood product transport and storage, which are relevant when considering temperature controls on board a blood delivery UAV.

Blood Product Storage and Transport Standards

To ensure its safe use during transfusion, blood must be transported and stored within particular temperature ranges as specified by the *Standards for Blood Banks and Transfusion Services* (AABB, 2018). Most relevant is Table Reference Standard 5.1.8A—Requirements for Storage, Transportation, and Expiration, which defines acceptable temperature ranges for a variety of blood products, including whole blood, RBCs, platelets, and plasma. For whole blood, nonfrozen RBCs, and thawed plasmas, the standards are consistently 1–6°C for storage and 1–10°C for transport. Transport and storage of platelets require temperatures between 20°C and 24°C, although platelets in storage also need continuous, gentle agitation to maintain product quality.

As will be discussed later in this chapter, the current consensus within the Joint medical community is that whole blood is the preferred product for transfusions to trauma patients in need of blood. It is unclear, however, which standard, storage or transport, applies to the emergency delivery of whole blood to injured personnel in the field, particularly if the blood is not transfused immediately. Based on discussions with researchers at the Army Institute of Surgical Research,[2] we apply the standard for storage, which states that whole blood must be maintained between 1°C and 6°C at all times prior to its use, even while on board a delivery platform or after being delivered to a forward position. Chapter Three discusses the implementation of a passive temperature control system (i.e., a cooler) that estimates the amount of insulation and coolant required to maintain blood within this 1–6°C temperature range during flight and post-delivery. Such systems, how-

---

[2]   Email communications with Joint medical community blood logisticians to understand blood transportation constraints, June 28–July 9, 2018.

ever, are not absolutely necessary. Zipline, for example, has not previously used cooling packs because delivery times have been short enough and an insulated wrap has been sufficient. Operations in the context of this analysis, however, are less certain; therefore, we assume relatively long post-delivery times without refrigeration or use.

Moving Blood with an Autonomous, Fixed-Wing UAV

As has been stated previously, this analysis assesses *autonomous, fixed-wing* UAVs for medical resupply. This section provides a brief overview of how we treat autonomy within this study and the inherent advantages of a fixed-wing platform. Delivery of blood by UAV also raises a more specific concern—namely, whether the quality of the product can be maintained throughout the duration of the flight. To address that issue, we briefly summarize studies that have assessed the impact of small UAV flights on blood quality.

Benefits of Autonomy and Fixed-Wing Aircraft

In general, the benefits of autonomous delivery are evident. Autonomous delivery helps to reduce logistical strain, as missions can be completed with minimal operator intervention, and helps to reduce risk associated with pilot error either en route or during delivery offload, assuming sufficient system reliability. More specifically, small UAVs are not necessarily constrained to operate from airfields, and their size implies relatively low unit costs, meaning more platforms can be more flexibly distributed throughout the theater. Within the context of this analysis, we consider autonomy only in terms of how it impacts the weight of the UAV, since the vehicle carries the necessary equipment, like radio frequency (RF) receivers and sensors, that enable pilotless flight. In this case, the model developed for the fleet design optimization analysis, discussed in Chapter Three, assumes that the total autonomous system electronics package is 0.2 kilogram.[3] Additional benefits

---

[3] This weight estimate is based on the Embention Veronte family of autopilots. See Embention (undated).

or disadvantages of autonomous delivery systems are beyond the scope of this study.

We also limit the scope of this analysis to strictly fixed-wing platforms. The terms *unmanned aircraft system* (UAS) and *drone* typically include quadcopters, but fixed-wing aircraft are inherently more efficient and typically capable of carrying larger payloads and traveling longer ranges. This fact can be observed from the range equation for a battery-powered, fixed-wing aircraft,

$$R = \eta_o \frac{L}{D} \frac{E_B}{W} ,$$

where R is the range, η_o is the overall efficiency of the vehicle, L/D is the lift-to-drag ratio (a measure of aerodynamic efficiency), E_b is the energy content of the battery, and W is the aircraft weight. For a fixed-wing aircraft, the lift-to-drag ratio is typically on the order of 10, while for a helicopter or a quadcopter, L/D is typically smaller. In addition, for a fixed-wing vehicle, all power drawn from the battery goes toward the forward motion of the aircraft, whereas for a helicopter some of that power must be used to keep the vehicle in the air, thus reducing the available energy for forward flight.[4]

Thus, because both lift-to-drag and effective battery energy content are higher, fixed-wing aircraft for the same range can carry more payload and for the same weight can travel a longer distance than a comparable helicopter or quadcopter. As will be shown in our definition of the notional blood delivery mission space, blood may require rapid transport over tens of miles, and thus we assume a priori that fixed-wing platforms are the most logical choice. This choice of configuration, however, does not rule out the future use of vertical takeoff and landing (VTOL) aircraft for similar missions if circumstances

---

[4]   While we will focus the analysis presented here on fixed-wing UAVs, there are other mission considerations that may drive the employment of a small rotary-wing asset. For example, delivery within the built vertical infrastructure of an urban area may drive the need for the greater maneuverability of a rotary-wing delivery vehicle. While range of a fixed-wing asset helps to scope the analysis presented here, it should be clear that a number of other operational factors can come into play to help inform the selection of UAV delivery assets.

were to require hover capability, either during takeoff, landing, or payload delivery.

It is worth noting that our analysis here does not take into account any requirements for equipment or infrastructure to launch or recover fixed-wing platforms. For example, the Zipline Zip utilizes a rail system for launch and a net apparatus for recovery of the asset. Factors such as cost and deployability of these assets, as well as any risk factors in the deployed environment, will play a role in the ultimate selection of the UAV delivery platform.

Does Small UAV Transport Degrade Blood Quality?

In addition to exposure to conditions above or below the required storage or transport temperature range, UAVs could also subject blood to accelerations and pressures that adversely affect its quality. Several studies have assessed the impact of low-altitude drone transport on the quality of whole blood (Amukele et al., 2015; Amukele et al., 2017). The authors of these studies tracked quality by comparing different indicators between a control (stationary samples) and samples that were flown on board fixed-wing platforms. Table 2.1 summarizes two flight tests performed by researchers at the Johns Hopkins University School of Medicine.

Researchers in both studies flew blood samples in fixed-wing platforms, cruising at 100 meters above ground level. Amukele et al. (2015) considered a relatively short flight of 30 minutes in a moderate ambient temperature of 25.3°C, with a UAV that was hand-launched. Amukele et al. (2017) assessed impacts from a longer three-hour flight in a hotter,

Table 2.1
Mission Parameters for Studies at the Johns Hopkins University School of Medicine

Study	Ambient Temp. (°C)	Range (km)	Altitude (m)	Flight Time (hrs)
Amukele et al. (2015)	25.3	40	100	0.5
Amukele et al. (2017)	32	260	100	3

SOURCES: Amukele et al., 2015; Amukele et al., 2017.

desert environment. This second study used a UAV capable of VTOL. For most blood quality indicators assessed, the two studies observed no statistically significant difference between the flown and control blood samples. The only exceptions were statistically significant differences in the potassium and glucose levels after the longer flight from Amukele et al. (2017). The research team hypothesized that this finding was related to the difference in storage temperatures between the two sets of samples. In both studies, temperature of the whole blood was not tightly maintained between 1°C and 6°C throughout the trials, thus violating blood storage standards, which potentially explains why potassium and glucose did not "meet clinical and/or regulatory acceptability criteria" applied in the study (Amukele et al., 2017).

Given the results of these analyses, we assume that transport on board a small UAV will not adversely impact the use of the whole blood in transfusions at MTFs or the point of injury as long as proper temperature controls are in place. These results, however, have not been proven robust under a variety of potential operating conditions and only extend to the combination of temperatures and accelerations assessed in the two flight tests, so we caution against the generalization of these results to other environmental and operational conditions. In addition, these results did not assess the impacts of reduced pressures on blood, as cruise altitudes were limited to 100 meters. At this altitude, pressures are within 1 percent of ground level. Future assessments could consider transport at reduced pressures, as higher cruise altitudes can correspond to higher flight vehicle efficiencies and reduced heat transfer requirements given the colder ambient temperatures. Subjecting samples to more extreme accelerations, comparable to maneuvers or hard landings that may be required in contested environments, may also be worthwhile.

Blood Transfusions and Improving Survival Outcomes

Intuition tells us that the sooner an injured person receives medical care, the better the odds that individual survives the injury. On average, this is indeed the case, where the Joint medical community has developed models, in particular the Joint Medical Planning Tool (JMPT),[5] to estimate these survival rates as a function of treatment timelines. JMPT survival curves then suggest that for traumatic injuries, where a person suffers substantial blood loss, starting blood transfusions and resuscitative care earlier (e.g., at the point of injury) can also potentially improve survival outcomes.

The literature on blood transfusions generally supports this conclusion. In particular, recent studies have assessed the benefits of prehospital transfusions on patient survival rates.[6] Shackelford et al. (2017) found that "blood product transfusion prehospital or within minutes of injury was associated with greater 24-hour and 30-day survival than delayed transfusion or no transfusion." More specifically, they observed that patients receiving prehospital transfusions experienced statistically significant reductions (approximately factor of three) in probability of death for both 24-hour and 30-day mortality. For the subset of patients who survived past 24 hours, however, the researchers did not observe a significant difference in outcomes. Within the subset of patients receiving transfusions, the researchers also observed statistically significant lower mortality rates for those receiving transfusions inside of 15 minutes than those receiving delayed transfusions.[7] Anecdotal evidence gathered through discussions with Joint medical community experts also supports the idea that earlier transfusions lead to better outcomes[8] and suggests a similar 15-minute ideal threshold from injury to start of transfusion.

Finally, we also note that the transfusion literature is also conclusive in one area—a balance between plasma, RBCs, and platelets leads to better outcomes than relying primarily on crystalloids such as

---

[5] JMPT assumes that patients receive blood as needed and thus cannot determine expected differences in survival outcomes with or without transfusions. For an overview of the JMPT methodology, we refer readers to Teledyne Brown Engineering Inc. (2015).

[6]   See, for example, Malsby et al. (2013), who implemented a prehospital transfusion process improvement initiative to ensure quality of care on board evacuation helicopters.

[7]   The average time to transfusion after injury in Shackelford et al. (2017) was 36 minutes.

[8]   Email communications with Joint medical community blood logisticians to understand blood transportation constraints, June 28–July 9, 2018.

saline during resuscitative care. Holcomb (2010), for example, found that 1:1:1 plasma-RBCs-platelets ratios led to improved outcomes. The military transfusion literature further concludes that whole blood is the preferred blood product for transfusions.[9] Specifying delivery of whole blood ultimately has little impact on this analysis because whole blood and blood components have similar storage temperature standards and mass densities (~1 gram/milliliter), the latter implying the weight and volume of the aircraft payload will not vary substantially with blood product type. This choice does, however, have broader logistical impacts that can determine what a UAV will carry on a given resupply or emergency delivery mission. We do not consider the precise logistical flows or demands of whole blood versus its components in this analysis.

Operating in a Contested or Denied Environment

Finally, the particular characteristics of a contested or denied environment have potentially significant consequences for the utility of autonomous UAVs. If an adversary denies RF transmissions, for example, then the system may not be able to receive GPS information. These data are sometimes used by the autopilot to correct errors that accumulate in inertial navigation systems on board unmanned aircraft. Without correction, these errors can lead to position drifts of hundreds or even thousands of meters over the course of a 10-mile or longer blood delivery mission.[10] There are, however, means to limit error accumulation even without GPS data. These methods include using predetermined environmental features or landmarks as well as other onboard

---

[9] See, for example, Cap et al. (2018), who state that "whole blood is the preferred product for resuscitation of severe traumatic hemorrhage. It contains all the elements of blood that are necessary for oxygen delivery and hemostasis, in nearly physiologic ratios and concentrations" (p. 44).

[10] Bryson and Sukkarieh (2004) give position errors for a small UAV assuming an uncorrected inertial navigation system.

sensors, like RADAR or LiDAR,[11] to help manage error buildup. These methods could be used to help mitigate the risk of off-target deliveries, particularly in emergency situations where time spent finding errant delivered payloads increases the risk to injured personnel in need of immediate medical attention. We do not consider the additional weight implications of these more capable navigation systems in this analysis.

Contested environments can also imply that systems are vulnerable to adversary tracking and targeting. One way to counter this situation is to fly as low as possible to take advantage of sensor horizon limitations and to minimize the distance a UAV might be within visual range. We incorporate this operational countermeasure into this analysis by specifying that all missions must be flown at low altitude—that is, we assume a mission pressure altitude, for vehicle sizing purposes, of zero meters.[12] Another counter to adversary sensors is to minimize the sensing cross-section of the platform, which is in part a function of the geometry and size of the aircraft. In this analysis we do not assess how this dependence might impact UAV design, but a sensing cross section model could potentially be implemented in future versions of the UAV design tool described in Chapter Three.

Another aspect of a high-threat, contested environment is the possibility that an adversary could employ conventional attacks to target the logistics support to UAV operations.[13] For example, should flight platforms require dedicated equipment such as rails and netting for their launch and recovery, an adversary may opt to target them with artillery or cruise missiles to degrade sortie generation capability at the

---

[11] See Kumar et al. (2017) for an example of a LiDAR/IMU navigation method for indoor UAVs. We also refer readers to the Simultaneous Localization and Mapping (SLAM) class of algorithms that researchers are developing specifically for GPS-denied environments.

[12] This does not account for any terrain, trees, or other environmental objects that could prevent a ground-hugging mission profile. As such, we do not consider the sensor or control package required for terrain avoidance and assume an ideal case where there are few obstructions along the UAV flight path. Future assessments can consider more refined mission profiles that more precisely define cruise altitudes for a given mission segment.

[13] For more on these threats to logistics support to flight operations, see Thomas et al., 2015.

site. Consequently, the high risk of a conventional threat to flight operations may drive the need for smaller UAV platforms with a reduced logistical footprint. While we do not account for these factors in this analysis, it should be clear that the nature of the threat environment will play an important role in the ultimate selection of the UAV platforms capable of accomplishing mission objectives.

The Blood Delivery Mission Space

We conclude this chapter by briefly outlining a notional mission space derived from the preceding discussion and which we use in Chapter Four to conduct the design optimization analysis. We define each mission within the space using three parameters: delivery range, the time in which the vehicle will need to make these deliveries, and the size of the single-trip payloads. All three of these parameters are a function of the type of mission, whether a logistical resupply or an emergency delivery.

Table 2.2 summarizes these parameters for both mission types. In this case, we assume that MTFs will be within 100 miles of each other,[14] while emergency deliveries will likely be to personnel operating approximately 10 miles away from the closest MTF (see Thomas et al., 2018, table 2.1). We assume delivery times for logistical resup-

Table 2.2
Summary of Mission Parameters for Logistical Resupply and Emergency Deliveries

Parameter	Logistical Resupply	Emergency Delivery
Range	~100 miles	~10 miles
Time	1 hour	15 minutes
Payload	10+ blood units	1 to 3 units

---

[14] Thomas et al. (2018) notes that theaterwide distribution of blood can exceed 100 miles, but we constrain the problem in this analysis to avoid excessively large vehicles.

ply missions to be on the order of one hour,[15] while UAVs will need to make emergency runs on the order of 15 minutes, which is a time derived from the transfusion literature previously summarized. Finally, we assume that resupplies will deliver 10 or more units of blood to replenish the stores at a small MTF,[16] while emergencies will require one to three units to treat one to three patients in the field.[17] If more units are required in either case, we assume it would be feasible to conduct additional, simultaneous deliveries. Finally, we note that users can customize these distances, response times, and payloads, allowing for analyses to be refined as necessary.

---

[15] We did not derive this quantity from the literature or expert elicitation, although it is loosely based on the Joint medical community's concept of the "golden hour."

[16] Thomas et al. (2018) specifies that a typical small MTF has enough refrigeration capacity for 30 units. Thus, a platform capable of delivering on the order of 10 units can replenish a large fraction of the small MTF's stores.

[17] We sized the emergency payload to be similar to the delivery capability of the Zipline UAVs—that is, payloads of one to three units (Thomas et al., 2018)—given the fundamentally similar on-demand, emergency operating concept. This range also corresponds to current military and civilian practices. For example, Zielinski et al. (2017) notes that Norwegian units typically carry two units of packed red blood cells (PRBCs) for emergency use. Also see McGinity et al. (2018) for an example of a civilian program in San Antonio that designates two units of whole blood for prehospital transfusion.

CHAPTER THREE

Rapid UAV Design Optimization of Fixed-Wing Fleets (RUDOFF) Model

This chapter describes the RUDOFF tool that we developed to design autonomous UAVs for blood delivery missions and estimate corresponding cost sensitivities.[1] This development was necessary, as existing UAV design tools had excessive computation times, unnecessary fidelity, or lack of capability tailored to small UAV design. First, we present a brief overview of UAV design optimization. Second, we discuss the specific optimization formulation applied to this problem—geometric programming (GP). Third, we summarize the primary components of RUDOFF. Finally, we present two model validation cases before applying the tool to the blood delivery mission space outlined in Chapter Four.

UAV Design Optimization

Design optimization of a UAV is similar to other optimization exercises—the vehicle obeys some set of physical laws, the mission space defines some set of performance constraints, and the goal is to minimize some quantity of interest relevant to the aircraft or mission.[2] Design of air vehicles can also present more specific challenges. First,

---

[1]   The RUDOFF tool we describe in this chapter focuses solely on the design parameters of the air vehicle itself. RUDOFF does not currently incorporate any logistical support requirements, such as the need for a specialized launch or recovery apparatus.

[2]   Weight (i.e., cost) is a common aircraft design optimization objective function.

they can be mixed-integer problems depending on the formulation (e.g., the wingspan can take a continuous value but there can only be an integer number of engines). Second, optimizers typically require reduced-order models to make problems computationally tractable, and thus some sacrifice in fidelity is commonly required. Developing these reduced-order models is also not always a trivial exercise.

Optimization techniques typically fall into two broad categories: (1) gradient-based approaches and (2) heuristics. Gradient-based methods rely on the calculation of either analytical or numerically estimated derivatives to minimize an objective (e.g., in a gradient-descent algorithm). The primary advantage of these methods is that they typically have provable convergence properties—you know you sit at a local minimum or maximum if the solution converges. Gradient methods, however, can be difficult to implement, particularly if the design space is not completely continuous. In addition, the ideal goal is to obtain globally optimal solutions (i.e., the best possible design for a given aircraft objective function); yet global optima are generally not guaranteed even if a gradient method converges.[3] As an example of a gradient-based tool, the Aircraft Concept Exploration System (ACES) developed here at RAND by Xu et al. (2016) uses sequential quadratic programming (SQP), an approximate gradient technique, to optimize aircraft designs.

The other set of approaches uses heuristics to move toward a design solution. These techniques are usually flexible (i.e., more easily implementable), can be used for mixed-integer problems, and do not require analytical or numerical estimates of gradients. The primary disadvantage, however, is that nothing can typically be said of the resulting "optimal" design other than it was the best conceived vehicle for a particular execution of the heuristic. Genetic algorithms (GAs) are popular in this space and have been used in a variety of aircraft conceptual design applications.[4] We will revisit GAs in the context of the UAV fleet design problem later in this report.

---

[3] If the optimization problem is convex, then convergence results in a globally optimal solution.

[4] See, for example, Antoine and Kroo (2005), who used genetic algorithms to explore aircraft design trade-offs between cost and environmental impact.

Geometric Programming

RUDOFF is a UAV design optimization tool built on the GP Python package, Gpkit (Burnell and Hoburg, 2018). Consider the following general optimization statement as given by Hoburg and Abbeel (2014),

$$\text{minimize } f_0(\boldsymbol{u})$$
$$\text{subject to } f_j(\boldsymbol{u}) \leq 1, \qquad i = 1, \ldots, m$$
$$h_j(\boldsymbol{u}) = 1, \qquad i = 1, \ldots, m_e,$$

where $\boldsymbol{u}$ is vector of free variables, f_0 is the objective function to be minimized, f_i are the inequality constraint functions, and h_j are the equality constraint functions. In the case of a UAV design optimization, $\boldsymbol{u}$ is the UAV design vector and functions f_i and h_j capture mission and vehicle constraints as well as the air vehicle physics. For an optimization problem to be a GP formulation, the following must be true: (1) f_0 and f_i must be *posynomial* functions and (2) h_j must be *monomial* functions. Posynomials are defined as polynomials with strictly positive coefficients and real-value exponents—for example, $2 + x^{0.482} y^{(-2)}$ is a posynomial where x and y are variables in the optimization. Monomials are single-term posynomials—for example, $x^{0.482} y^{(-2)}$. As a counterexample, $1 - 2xy^3$ is neither a posynomial nor a monomial.

This formulation has two key advantages. First, given the defined functional forms, performing a logarithmic transformation creates a convex optimization problem.[5] This is most easily observed for the monomial equality constraints—taking the log of both sides yields a linear relationship, which is a convex function. This means that a GP problem is guaranteed to yield a globally optimal solution. Second, convex problems are readily solved by current optimization packages, leading to fast solution times.[6]

The disadvantage, however, is that this formulation is restrictive because all physical laws or reduced-order models need to be cast

---

[5]   As proof of function convexity, we refer the reader to Boyd et al. (2007).

[6]   The optimizer, Mosek, implemented within GPkit uses an interior-point method for non-linear convex optimization problems.

as GP-compatible functions (i.e., posynomials and monomials). This then begs the question: Can we solve useful problems using geometric programming? GP formulations were first proposed for conceptual aircraft design by Hoburg and Abbeel (2014), who showed that indeed aircraft design first principles sufficient for early conceptual design analysis could be captured with these types of functions. The next section describes how we improve on and extend the Hoburg and Abbeel (2014) model to optimize small UAVs for delivery missions.

RUDOFF Overview

RUDOFF builds off the work of Hoburg and Abbeel (2014)[7] and incorporates elements specific to small UAV design and blood delivery missions. It has two primary components: (1) an inner model built on the Python library GPkit and (2) an outer model that searches for the optimal fleet design, given a specified number of desired platforms. Here we describe both the inner and outer model in greater detail and how they are integrated. We also provide brief overviews of the blood payload and UAV cost models as these may be of interest to readers. Finally, we also developed a corresponding visualization tool that is described in Appendix C.

Inner Model: GPkit Optimization

The inner model, which we will interchangeably refer to as the "GP model," is an extension of the work in Hoburg and Abbeel (2014) and performs the UAV design optimization that is ultimately used by the outer model to select the design of the single-platform or multiplatform fleet. Figure 3.1 shows the components of the inner model, which we built with an object-oriented structure. As shown, the model is composed of two primary objects: *Aircraft* and *Mission Flier*. These two objects take a set of user-defined inputs that determine certain characteristics of the UAV (e.g., electric- or gas-powered) and the mission space (e.g., range, payload) for which the UAV design is optimized.

---

[7]   Note that a "model" in this sense is defined by a set of GP-compatible inequality and/or equality constraints that capture the physics or relationships of interest.

Figure 3.1
Structure and Components of the Inner (GP) Model

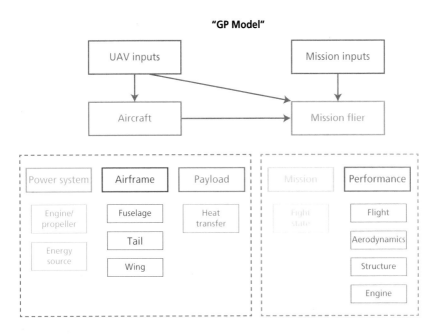

The *Aircraft* object defines the physical UAV that consists of the power system, airframe, and payload. The power system is defined by the thrust-generating mechanism and the energy source. In this analysis, the thrust generator is always assumed to be a single propeller powered by either an internal-combustion engine or electric motor. The energy source is then either a hydrocarbon fuel or lithium-ion batteries, respectively. The airframe is composed of the fuselage, tail, and wing, with the corresponding models capturing the shape and weight of each component. The weight of the payload is either user-defined or, in the case of blood delivery, estimated from the number of blood units and the corresponding amount of coolant and insulation needed to keep the blood within the whole blood standard temperature range of 1°C to 6°C, as discussed previously in Chapter Two.

The *Mission Flier* object, as implied by the name, flies the *Aircraft* on the user-defined set of missions. *Mission Flier* has two primary elements. First, a mission model tracks the different flight states (speed, altitude, etc.) of the UAV as it executes its mission. Second, several performance models ensure that the UAV obeys physical laws. These include constraints requiring flight equilibrium and sufficient structural strength as well as sets of functions that define the aerodynamic performance of the wing and tail and the efficiency of the engine and propeller, among others.

As will be discussed in more detail when we explain the outer model, multiple missions can be assigned to a single *Aircraft* object, although a *Mission Flier* object captures only a single mission. Thus, the number of *Mission Flier* objects that are created reflect the number of missions a user assigns to a given UAV. The user then specifies an objective function of interest, which can be a function of the variables defined within an *Aircraft* object or any number of the relevant *Mission Flier* objects. When the optimization solver is called, two outcomes are possible: (1) a feasible UAV design that reflects the global minimum value of the objective function or (2) an infeasible solution (i.e., a UAV design does not exist that satisfies all of the specified constraints). We discuss the consequences of an infeasible solution as it pertains to the fleet design problem below.

The GP model has been specifically developed for small UAV design analysis and, as shown later in this section, has only been validated against this class of air vehicles.[8] As discussed in Chapter One, small UAVs correspond to DoD Groups 1 and 2 (U.S. Army, 2010). Small UAV performance is distinctly different from the performance of larger aircraft as the aerodynamics, in some ways, are more challenging. We built the aerodynamics models to specifically account for the flight regimes more commonly associated with smaller aircraft.[9] In addition, the weight model is likely only valid for small UAVs given the assumed empirical scaling with geometry.

---

[8]   Hoburg and Abbeel (2014) do not explicitly address to which scale their model most readily applies, although their example is for a Group 4/5-sized aircraft.

[9]   These are typically referred to as *low Reynolds number* flight regimes. The airfoil assumed in this analysis is not optimized for this kind of flight.

Appendix A discusses more of the technical details of the inner model, but we highlight two of the submodels in greater detail in the next two subsections. Appendix B provides a summary of user-definable inputs for a given analysis.

Blood Payload Model

As summarized in Chapter Two, blood must be stored within a certain temperature range. Discussion with Army blood logisticians suggested that these standards would not be relaxed for blood transport on small UAVs during emergency deliveries or logistical shipments or while blood is being carried in the field post-delivery.[10] Thus the onboard payload must also include the weight of the temperature control system.

For simplicity, we assume that a cooler provides passive temperature control and has two components: (1) insulation and (2) a phase change material (PCM). Insulation restricts heat flow across the boundary of the cooler while the PCM stores or releases energy based on the difference between the internal and external temperatures.[11] We estimate the weight of these two components within the blood payload model using heat transfer first principles. The weight of the insulation is a function of the difference in temperature between the mission environment and the optimal temperature range for blood—this sets the heat flux into or out of the cooler and the volume required to store the blood. The weight of the PCM is a function of how much energy storage capacity is required. This in turn is a function of the heat flux into or out of the box, the PCM heat of fusion (i.e., melting point), and the PCM's specific heat capacity. The total payload weight is then the sum of the blood product, insulation, and PCM weights.

We validate the blood payload model by comparing the estimated weight to the weight of the Golden Hour Medic Series 4 from Pelican BioThermal.[12] The Medic Series 4 reports for "optimal conditions,"

---

[10] Email communications with Joint medical community blood logisticians to understand blood transportation constraints, June 28–July 9, 2018.

[11] During blood transport, wet ice is the most common PCM for liquid products and dry ice for frozen products. Other commercially produced PCMs are available for specialized temperature ranges specific to cold chain management (Thomas et al., 2018).

[12] See Pelican BioThermal (2017) for cooling performance data sheets.

assumed here to correspond to a 15°C temperature difference between the ambient environment and the cooler, that blood can be stored between 2°C and 8°C for 72 hours. Using those parameters in the RUDOFF blood payload, we estimate that a cooler that meets these specifications would weigh approximately 7.5 pounds, where reported Medic Series 4 weights are between seven and 10 pounds.

UAV Unit-Cost Model

We estimate UAV unit cost using the model developed by Valerdi (2005), who proposed two cost-estimating relationships (CERs) for UAVs. The first is a linear relationship given by

$$C = \$400 \text{ per Newton} \times W_{ew}, \tag{1}$$

where C is the unit cost and W_{ew} is the empty weight[13] of the UAV in Newtons.[14] The second relates unit cost to the payload weight times vehicle endurance. For the aircraft sizes considered in this analysis, the two CERs produce similar cost estimates; thus, for the sake of simplicity, we use Equation (1) in our model. We note that these results are based on a relatively small number of data points and may not reflect current achievable UAV unit costs. In addition, this CER is likely only valid for projecting future costs of similar UAVs (i.e., those with similar materials, propulsions systems, and flight control packages). Future work should look to improve these UAV CERs by, for example, adding corrections for advanced materials or other next-generation technologies.

Outer Model: Fleet Design Search

The outer model interacts with the inner model to generate an optimized fleet design for a given application. We formulate the fleet design search as a combinatorial optimization problem, as illustrated in Figure

---

[13] Empty weight is defined as the aircraft weight without fuel or cargo.

[14] Note that this estimate underestimates the actual reported unit cost of the RQ-11B, while other RAND UAV CERs overestimate this unit cost. Both approaches, however, use aircraft empty weight as the independent variable.

3.2. A user defines N missions and would like K aircraft to fly all or, if not feasible, a subset of those missions. The goal of the outer model is then to optimally assign as many of those N missions to the K aircraft based on a fleet objective function (FOF) set by the user.[15]

We define the FOF, in general, to have two elements. The first reflects some aspect of the UAV design that the user wishes to optimize (which can also serve as the objective for the GP model call). For example, this could be to minimize the life-cycle cost of a given platform. The second is some measure of how much the K UAVs span the defined mission space. An example FOF could be

$$\text{FOF} = \left(\sum\nolimits_{i=1}^{K} \alpha_i C_i \right)^{-1} + \sum\nolimits_{j=1}^{N} \beta_j x_j, \tag{2}$$

where the first term represents a weighted fleet cost and the second is a weighted term that captures the number of missions assigned to the UAVs with x_j taking values of 0 or 1.[16] Note that the first term is inversely proportional to cost such that the FOF places more value on lower cost platforms (i.e., the FOF decreases with increasing cost).[17] We also note that in the following applications of this objective function, we implement the second FOF term such that a given mission can only be assigned to a single UAV, as reflected in Figure 3.2. This is also likely the lowest-cost case because redundant capability across multiple platforms can only increase total life-cycle costs. More generally, however, some redundancy may be desired. For example, a critical mission may exist that all platforms in the fleet must be able to execute.

---

[15] Because the fleet optimization problem only calls the GP model, the FOF does not need to be GP-compatible.

[16] Not all missions can or will be assigned. For example, if the addition of a particular mission generates an infeasible result when the inner model is called, then the FOF would be passed a large negative value, making it effectively impossible for that mission allocation to be selected.

[17] It is also common practice to normalize all quantities in the FOF so as to avoid issues with conflicting scales and units. This normalization is inherent in the analysis presented later in this report.

Figure 3.2
Illustration of the Fleet Search Problem for *N* = 4, *K* = 2

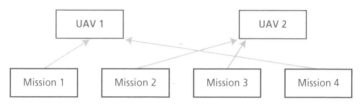

NOTE: In this case, Mission 1 and Mission 4 have been assigned to UAV 1, while Mission 2 and Mission 3 have been assigned to UAV 2.

For simplicity, we do not consider this particular case in Chapter Four, but we note that the FOF in RUDOFF could be defined to require such redundancy. The fleet design search then seeks to maximize this example FOF by simultaneously minimizing cost and maximizing the mission space coverage.[18]

The cost function can also be broken down into multiple components. In this analysis, we assume that aircraft cost includes the one-time cost to develop the system, the cost of procurement (i.e., number of procured units times unit cost), and recurring sustainment costs over the course of the system's lifetime. We can then write the cost of aircraft i as

$$C_i = C_{i,D} + n_{\text{units}} \cdot C_{i,U} + n_m \cdot n_{\text{units}} \cdot C_{i,m} , \qquad (3)$$

where $C_{i,D}$ is the development cost, n_{units} is the total number of acquired units, $C_{i,U}$ is the unit cost, n_m is the number of missions flown over the course of the system lifetime per unit, and $C_{i,m}$ is the cost per flown mission. The cost per flown mission can include costs directly related to the mission (e.g., fuel) and required maintenance. In the validation case presented in Appendix A, as well as the simple fleet optimization for a blood delivery UAV fleet in Chapter Four, we assume that $C_{i,m}$

---

[18] Conversely, a FOF could be defined such that the search algorithm would seek to minimize its value.

Figure 3.3
How the Outer Model Interacts with the Inner (GP) Model
to Update the FOF and Ultimately Generate an "Optimal"
Fleet Design

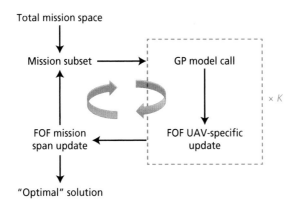

only captures mission-related costs that are proportional to the energy consumed during execution of the mission.

Figure 3.3 illustrates how the outer model is structured around the GP model. For a given mission space, the fleet design search iterates through possible mission allocations to the specified number of UAVs, and we refer to a given mission allocation as a *mission subset*. Within each mission subset, the inner model is called K times to calculate the corresponding UAV-specific element of the FOF. Then, once the inner model function calls are complete, the routine updates the FOF with the mission-spanning factor—that is, the second term in Equation (2) for the given mission subset. These iterations are carried out until a specified stopping criterion is met.

An exhaustive search of all possible mission subsets, in general, is not feasible. For instance, there can be billions of unique mission assignment combinations for reasonably sized problems (e.g., four aircraft and 20 missions). For the cases considered in this analysis, a genetic algorithm is used to select the "optimal" mission subset. Appendix A provides more detail of the specific implementation of the GA.

Model Validation

We present two validation cases for the GP model. The first is the AeroVironment RQ-11B Raven, used for short-range intelligence gathering. The second is the Zipline Zip 1, which has been used for blood delivery between medical facilities in Rwanda. The purpose of these validation cases is to show that RUDOFF, including its underlying simplifications, generates accurate results for small UAVs and can be confidently applied to similar but novel problems. As will be seen for the RQ-11B, deviations between model outputs and actual UAV parameters are small but are unavoidable given RUDOFF's low fidelity and our approximately defined mission sets based on publicly reported capability. Appendix A also offers a validation of the outer fleet optimization model using a randomly generated mission space.

Validation Case 1: AeroVironment RQ-11B Raven

Figure 3.4 shows the AeroVironment RQ-11B Raven, an autonomous, battery-powered, low-altitude intelligence, surveillance, and reconnaissance (ISR) UAV for military applications. From the Raven data sheet, the mission space is defined by a range of 10 kilometers (km), an endurance between 60 and 90 minutes, operating speeds between 8.9 and 22.5 meters/second (m/s), and operating altitudes between 30 and 152 meters above ground level (AGL) (AeroVironment, 2017b). From these specifications, we defined the RQ-11B mission space to include three missions for which we optimize the vehicle design:

- Mission 1: fly out 10 km at 22.5 m/s, loiter for 1 hour at 15 m/s, fly back 10 km at 22.5 m/s.
- Mission 2: fly out 10 km at 14 m/s, loiter for 1.5 hours at 10 m/s, fly back 10 km at 14 m/s.
- Mission 3: fly out 10 km at 8.9 m/s, fly back 10 km at 8.9 m/s.

We selected these missions to both span the defined performance bounds and pose realistic operational scenarios. For example, the first two profiles might be longer-endurance surveillance missions while the third might be a tracking mission.

Figure 3.4
AeroVironment RQ-11B Raven: An Autonomous, Low-Altitude ISR UAV

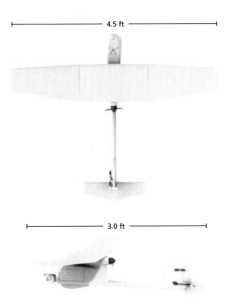

SOURCE: AeroVironment, 2017a, used with permission.
NOTE: ISR = intelligence, surveillance, and reconnaissance.

We define the objective function in this case to be a trade-off between two vehicle characteristics: battery weight and wing aspect ratio. Minimizing battery weight is similar to the objective of minimizing aircraft weight and thus cost—the lighter the vehicle, the less required power for flight. We select battery weight instead, however, because it also has logistical implications—the less battery on board, the lower the recharge time and the quicker the vehicle turnaround. Wing aspect ratio, which is defined as the square of the wingspan divided by the wing planform area, can be thought of as a geometric complexity factor. A higher aspect ratio corresponds to a larger wingspan, which complicates manufacturing and increases the physical footprint of the vehicle, making it harder to transport and safely store. A lower aspect ratio, however, corresponds to reduced aerodynamic efficiency, leading to more power required for flight for a given aircraft weight. Thus, the two factors create a natural trade-off.

Figure 3.5
Visual Comparison Between RUDOFF Output and RQ-11

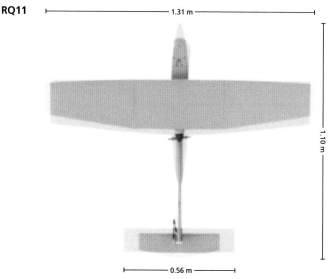

SOURCES: AeroVironment, 2017a, used with permission; RUDOFF tool.

With both the objective function and mission set defined, the GP model generates a set of globally optimal designs based on different weightings of the battery weight and wing aspect ratio terms. For the nominal weighting case (e.g., the two terms are weighted approximately equally), Figure 3.5 plots the comparison between the model output and the actual RQ-11B. We can see that the RUDOFF output achieves good agreement with the physical dimensions of the RQ-11B. Table 3.1 compares the actual RQ-11B specifications to those gener-

Table 3.1
Comparison of RUDOFF Outputs and RQ-11B Actuals for the RQ-11B Validation Case

	Wingspan (m)	Chord (m)	Weight (kg)
Actual	1.37	0.22	1.9
RUDOFF	1.31	0.25	1.9

ated by the GP model for this nominal case, where we can see that model outputs are within approximately 5 to 20 percent of the actuals for the three presented parameters.

Figure 3.6 shows the resulting Pareto front when considering trade-offs between wing aspect ratio and battery weight, where we provide visualizations for the two bounding cases. Not surprisingly, as the

Figure 3.6
Pareto Trade-Off Between Battery Weight and Wing Aspect Ratio

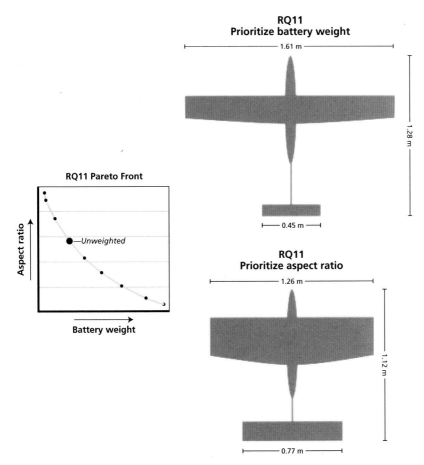

SOURCE: RUDOFF tool.
NOTE: We do not plot units on the Pareto chart. However, observe the direction of increasing aspect ratio and battery weight.

aspect ratio term is weighted more heavily, the shorter and stubbier the wings become. Figure 3.6 also highlights the usefulness of performing such a trade space analysis. Any one of the designs indicated along the curve can perform the set of defined missions (i.e., RUDOFF converged for each unique definition of the objective function coupled with the model and mission constraints). Depending on what stakeholders more highly value, however, this curve also shows that the current RQ-11B design (marked "Unweighted" on the curve) is perhaps not the optimal design when considering battery weight or aspect ratio; that is, the RQ-11B could be more optimally redesigned along either of these dimensions and still operate within our defined mission space. Each design point, however, will have a different associated cost, allowing analysts to visualize relevant design trade-offs and their impact on program cost.

Validation Case 2: Zipline Zip 1

We also performed a validation case comparing GP model outputs to the Zipline Zip 1, the first-generation autonomous, battery-powered UAV deployed by Zipline for blood delivery in Rwanda.[19] We assume a similar objective function as for the RQ-11, weighting the battery mass and wing aspect ratio terms approximately equally, and define a single mission based on stated Zip 1 mission capability—fly out 80 kilometers at 70 kilometers/hour (km/h) or 19.4 m/s, deliver payload, fly back 80 km at 70 km/h (Stewart, 2017). This case differs from the RQ-11B case as the UAV is now lighter on the return leg of its flight after payload delivery.

Table 3.2 compares the GP model outputs and the Zip 1 actuals. The GP model outputs are not consistent with the Zip 1 specifications, as the GP-model-generated UAV is both lighter and smaller. Given the similarity between the RQ-11B and Zip 1 in both payload, capable cruise speed, and total ground distance covered (i.e., when the distance covered during loiter is accounted for with the Raven), the Zip 1 is still approximately six times heavier than the Raven. This suggests three possible explanations for the discrepancies between the model

---

[19] For an overview of the Zipline platform and business model, see Zipline (undated).

Table 3.2
Comparison of GP Model Outputs with Actuals for the Zipline Zip 1 UAV Validation Case

	Wingspan (m)	Chord (m)	Weight (kg)
Actual	1.83	0.24	12–14
GP Model	1.67	0.29	8.7
GP Model–Matched	1.89	0.28	12.7

SOURCES: RUDOFF tool; Stewart, 2017.

and actual specifications for the Zipline UAV: (1) It is overengineered relative to constraints in the model, thus increasing vehicle weight;[20] (2) it is more capable than the missions it flies, perhaps having the ability to fly longer-range missions or carry more payload; (3) there are more components on board than captured in this model. If, for example, we artificially force the model to match the weight of the actual Zip 1 (see GP Model–Matched in Table 3.2), the model more accurately reproduces the dimensions of the UAV. Future model development should prioritize improving the UAV weight and structural models within RUDOFF.[21]

Comparing Computational Performance with ACES

Finally, we also compare the computational performance of RUDOFF to RAND's current aircraft conceptual design tool, ACES, to highlight the benefits of a GP approach. For a 200 variable problem, RUDOFF computes the optimal UAV design in approximately 1 second—about 0.9 second to initialize the model run and 0.1 second for the GPkit model to solve. ACES, by comparison, takes approximately 5 minutes

---

[20] This is certainly feasible given that the UAV has to withstand the end of the mission capture system, a hook that decelerates and catches the aircraft. The GP model structural model does not account for these stresses on the airframe, thus likely underestimating the structural weight.

[21] As stated in Chapter One, Zipline has since deployed the Zip 2, a larger and more capable platform with a reported 80-miles-per-hour (mph) cruise speed that can deliver a 1.75 kg payload (Petrova and Koldony, 2018). The GP model similarly underestimates the vehicle weight and dimensions of the Zip 2.

to solve a similarly sized problem, which is a difference of two orders of magnitude. We note, however, that ACES is a higher-fidelity model that allows for more general aircraft design optimization and thus in many cases warrants the longer computation times (Xu et al., 2016). RUDOFF is specifically designed for small UAV analyses and makes several assumptions regarding aircraft configuration to simplify the model implementation. RUDOFF should be viewed as a preliminary design tool whose optimized design outputs can then be refined by ACES.

CHAPTER FOUR

Design of an Autonomous UAV Fleet for Blood Delivery

The previous chapters outlined the utility of an autonomous delivery UAV for blood resupply and defined the mission space in which the vehicle may operate. We specify two primary functions: (1) to resupply MTFs with blood to provide additional logistical flexibility and (2) to perform emergency delivery of whole blood to injured personnel at forward-operating locations. This chapter uses RUDOFF, described and validated in Chapter Three, to optimize the design of a blood delivery UAV given the defined mission space. First, we assess a one-size-fits-all solution—that is, we design a single platform that serves both functions. We then perform a sensitivity analysis to understand the most important UAV design drivers. Second, we consider a fleet consisting of multiple platforms. As will be seen, this exercise amounts to optimizing two aircraft designs, one for each function. We then compare these designs to the one-size-fits-all solution. Finally, we conclude with a brief discussion of the acquisition implications of a single-platform versus multiplatform fleet.

Optimizing a One-Size-Fits-All Small UAV

This section optimizes the design of a one-size-fits-all UAV that resupplies MTFs and delivers emergency whole blood to forward operators. Based on the notional mission space (defined at the end of Chapter Two), Table 4.1 gives the precise range, speed, and payload parameters

Table 4.1
Precise Range, Time, and Payload Parameter Definitions
for the One-Size-Fits-All UAV Optimization

Parameter	Logistical Resupply	Emergency Delivery
Range	100 miles	25 miles
Time	1.5 hours	15 minutes
Payload	10 blood units	2 units

Table 4.2
Heat Transfer Parameters to Size Blood Payload

Parameter	Logistical Resupply	Emergency Delivery
Storage time	3 hours	72 hours
Temperature difference	15°C	15°C

applied in the optimization. In addition, Table 4.2 lists the parameters we used to design the blood cooler to meet storage standards. The assumed temperature difference is meant to approximately reflect a standard atmosphere at ground.

We define the objective function to be the estimated life-cycle cost of the aircraft as described in Equation (3) in Chapter Three, similar to the objective used in the fleet optimization validation case in Appendix A. To estimate this cost, we assume a 10-unit fleet in which each unit will ultimately fly a total of 1,000 logistical resupply missions and make 100 emergency deliveries over the course of the fleet lifetime.[1] We estimate unit costs using Equation (1). Multiplying this value by the fleet size gives the total procurement costs.[2] Development costs are

---

[1]   We arbitrarily selected the fleet size and mission frequencies; these parameters are easily modified to reflect actual program requirements.

[2]   CERs can include adjustments for different aircraft lot sizes and cumulative learning curve effects. The more aircraft manufactured in a given year and overall typically corresponds to lower average unit costs. See, for example, Younossi et al. (2001). We do not account for these and other learning effects, although they can be incorporated in the future with GP-compatible objective functions.

then assumed to be 100 times the unit cost.[3] Finally, we estimate mission energy costs assuming $0.20 per kilowatt-hour (kWh), which is close to the global average cost of electricity per kilowatt-hour.[4]

Figure 4.1 also gives the resulting optimized design of the one-size-fits-all UAV. The aircraft has a wingspan of 1.92 meters with a battery weight of 25.3 kilograms and a total takeoff weight of 51.5 kg. The total energy costs to fly each mission using the single platform are 4.2 kWh and 1.1 kWh for the logistical resupply and emergency delivery missions, respectively. As mentioned previously, we have assumed that this small UAV will be battery-powered, as similar-sized aircraft such as the Zip 1 and RQ-11B are powered by electric propulsion systems. Using RUDOFF, however, we can also consider a gas-powered UAV. Given the higher specific energy of hydrocarbon fuels, an optimized gas-powered design is, not surprisingly, lighter, with a total takeoff weight of 16.5 kg. The mission energy costs, however, are now 5.7 kWh and 1.4 kWh, respectively, given the less efficient combustion engines. The difference in life-cycle costs between similarly sized gas-powered and electric UAVs, however, are less certain and will be a function of maintenance requirements: While electric aircraft may be cheaper to maintain compared to internal combustion engines,[5] finite battery lifetimes may ultimately limit these benefits. Future work should perform more detailed assessments of differences in life-cycle costs for gas- versus electric-powered small UAVs.

Assessing Design Sensitivities of the One-Size-Fits-All UAV

RUDOFF also generates sensitivity information—that is, the percentage change in the objective function given a percentage change in one

---

[3]   We derived this estimate from aircraft selected acquisition reports (SARs), where total program development costs were typically two orders of magnitude greater than the average unit cost.

[4]   Average electricity costs in the United States are approximately $0.12/kWh (EIA, 2018). We round up to $0.20/kWh assuming that it will be inherently more expensive to generate electricity at operational locations.

[5]   Electric motors are simpler than their mechanical counterparts. Lower maintenance costs have been cited as one of the potential benefits of electric aviation. See, for example, Bye (2017).

of the design or mission input parameters. This information is available for all model parameters, as GPkit uses them to solve the UAV design optimization problem. These data are useful for users to understand how sensitive, for example, life-cycle costs might be to different assumptions regarding the mission space.

Figure 4.1 also provides a tornado plot of the expected percentage change in the previously defined life-cycle cost given a percent change in the corresponding mission space parameter. As we can see, the life-cycle cost is most sensitive to the minimum range[6] defined for the logistical resupply mission. In this case, we would expect that an aircraft that is capable of flying at least 150 miles (i.e., a 50-percent increase) would increase total life-cycle costs by 70 percent. Costs are also sensitive to the size of the logistical resupply payload, where one additional payload unit (i.e., a 10-percent increase in payload size) would increase total life-cycle costs by approximately 6 percent, given aircraft weight, and thus mission energy costs increase. In both of these examples, cost is less sensitive to the minimum range and number of units in the payload for the emergency delivery mission, indicating that the logistical resupply mission is the primary cost driver of the one-size-fits-all platform. Finally, we note that costs are less sensitive to the specified response time for each mission. In fact, costs are nearly insensitive to the logistical resupply response time while a 10-percent decrease in the emergency response time corresponds to a 0.8-percent increase in life-cycle costs. Note that the sensitivities are negative, since a decrease in response time implies a higher minimum cruise velocity, thus requiring more power delivered to the aircraft.

With these sensitivities, program officials can estimate the cost of additional capability, as highlighted above. In the increased range example, a 150-mile-capable UAV would cost approximately $5.5 million more over the course of the lifetime of the single-platform fleet using our previously defined total life-cycle cost. Note, however, that

---

[6] Note that the mission range constraint is applied as a "minimum." That is, the UAV must fly at least the distance specified in Table 2.2, but could fly farther if so specified by the optimization. For minimum cost configurations, however, a UAV typically did not fly any farther than specified by the mission constraints.

Figure 4.1
Illustration of Optimal Design and Cost Sensitivities (Percent Change in Life-Cycle Cost for a 1-Percent Change in Mission Parameter) for the "One-Size-Fits-All" UAV

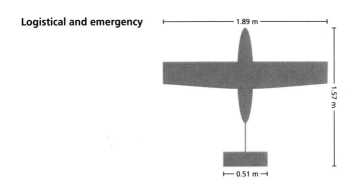

Logistical and emergency

1.89 m

1.57 m

0.51 m

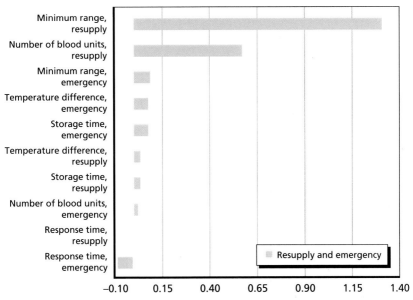

Sensitivities: One Size Fits All

SOURCE: RUDOFF tool.

such an increase in range may ultimately yield an infeasible optimization problem (i.e., no aircraft can be designed that meets this set of mission requirements). Issues regarding feasible designs cannot be observed from the sensitivities. Instead, RUDOFF would have to be executed again with the new mission added to the mission space to be sure a capable UAV exists.

Visualizing Objective Function Trade-Offs

The optimal design generated in the previous section did not include a design complexity factor (e.g., the aspect ratio term from the RQ-11B validation case). We can, however, still consider different weightings of the terms in the estimated life-cycle cost objective function. For example, if operators anticipate flying these UAVs in relatively austere environments where they may be limited in their ability to recharge the vehicle batteries, then designs with lower energy costs may be more highly valued. Alternatively, acquisition officials may prioritize a cheaper development phase and lower unit procurement cost while being less concerned with higher mission costs.

Figure 4.2 shows the optimal Pareto curve that considers trade-offs between normalized unit and development versus mission energy costs. Three points are plotted; moving from the upper left to lower right corresponds to increasing emphasis on lower development and unit costs at the expense of higher mission energy. The two visualizations, moving from top to bottom, show the corresponding optimal UAV designs at the two indicated bounding points. As energy costs are less heavily weighted relative to development and unit costs, the corresponding changes in aircraft geometry follow from fundamental aircraft design principles. For example, larger wingspans are typically associated with lower (induced) drag and slower missions and thus lower energy use. Given how we defined life-cycle cost, however, this corresponds to a heavier aircraft, and thus higher development[7] and unit costs. Moving down and to the right on the curve, however, leads to smaller wingspan aircraft, corresponding to lower development/unit costs but higher energy costs as the UAV must now fly more quickly and/or operate at a higher lift coefficient. For the plotted cases,

---

[7]   We refer to this as research, development, test, and evaluation (RDT&E) in Figure 4.2.

Figure 4.2
Pareto Trade-Off Between RDT&E + Unit Costs Versus Mission Energy Costs, Including Visualizations for Each Plotted Point

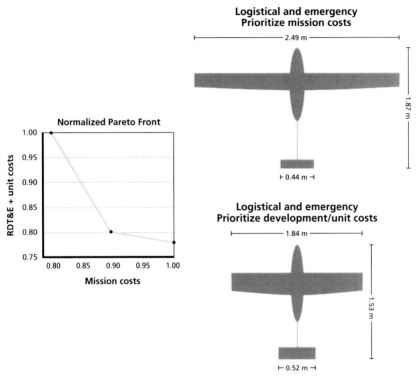

SOURCE: RUDOFF tool.
NOTE: RDT&E = research, development, test, and evaluation.

a 25-percent reduction in total unit and development costs leads to a 30-percent increase in total lifetime mission energy costs.

Finally, we note that the mission energy costs are small (on the order of 1 percent) compared with the development and total procurement cost. Real acquisition programs, however, have expensive sustainment phases, and capturing additional costs such as maintenance cycles and part replacement can change the trade-offs along this Pareto front and lead to different optimal designs for a given weighting between the two cost terms. Future analyses should develop and implement more detailed cost functions to capture all relevant small UAV program elements.

Comparing the One-Size-Fits-All Platform to Existing UAVs

We conclude our analysis of the one-size-fits-all solution by comparing its design to existing UAV platforms. Table 4.3 provides the high-level design specifications for the one-size-fits-all blood delivery UAV, RQ-11B Raven, and Zipline Zip 1. As we can see, the one-size-fits-all platform is distinct from both the RQ-11B and Zip 1. With regard to the Raven, our optimized blood delivery UAV is both larger and heavier, driven by the two orders of magnitude greater payload requirement, greater range and endurance requirement of the logistical resupply mission, and the power requirements of the faster emergency delivery mission. With regard to the Zip 1, the overall physical dimensions are similar, but the payload requirements are different, leading to an almost twice as heavy optimized design. This result highlights the fact that not all UAVs are equally capable and different mission sets may require wholly different platforms. Specifically, for blood delivery missions, this comparison suggests that the RQ-11B may be inadequate to serve Joint medical community needs, particularly for longer-range logistical resupply tasks, given the Raven's mission radius.[8]

Table 4.3
High-Level Design Specifications of the RQ-11B Raven, Zipline Zip 1, the One-Size-Fits-All Platform, and the Two Mission-Specific Platforms

Platform	Wingspan (m)	Chord (m)	Weight (kg)	Payload (kg)
RQ-11B Raven	1.37	0.22	1.9	0.2
Zip 1	1.83	0.24	12–14	1.5[a]
One-Size-Fits-All	1.89	0.33	39.9	10
Logistical	1.86	0.32	37.0	10
Emergency	1.07	0.23	17.7	9.1

SOURCES: AeroVironment, 2017b; RUDOFF tool; Stewart, 2017.
[a] Authors' estimate.

---

[8]   In a more extreme example, this result also implies that the larger-class UAVs, such as the MQ-9 Reaper, are larger and faster than what is necessary for blood delivery missions. This highlights the other end of the spectrum—namely, the minimum capability that is required that offers the necessary mission flexibility constrained by the fact that larger systems typically cost more.

This is not to say that existing platforms cannot serve other purposes. Future RUDOFF development could focus on a mission set feasibility analyzer; that is, given the characteristics of an existing platform, the model would fly a set of user-defined missions to determine if the existing platform can provide that mission capability. This would allow stakeholders and acquisition program officials of existing systems to understand how they can better use current fleets.

Mission-Specific UAV Platforms

The previous sections assessed the one-size-fits-all solution (i.e., a fleet with multiple units of a single UAV platform flying both mission types). In this section, we now turn our attention to a multiplatform fleet. Consider, for example, that operators have elected to use a unique platform for each mission type, whereby one UAV type flies the logistical resupply missions while a second platform makes the emergency deliveries. In this case, the objective is then to minimize the life-cycle costs of both platforms for their respective mission space.

Figure 4.3 gives the optimized design for each mission. We see that the logistical resupply UAV is similar in size to the one-size-fits-

Figure 4.3
Visualizations of the Mission-Specific Platforms: Logistical Resupply UAV (Left); Emergency Delivery UAV (Right)

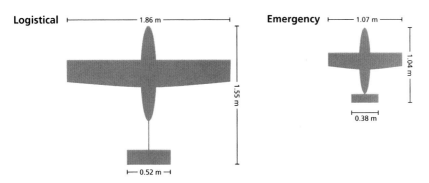

SOURCE: RUDOFF tool.

all solution while the emergency delivery aircraft is about 40 percent smaller, as reported in Table 4.3. This result follows, given that in both missions the payloads are actually of similar size and weight but the range requirements of the logistical mission demands a larger aircraft capable of carrying a larger battery for its longer mission. The mission-specific UAVs also expend different amounts of energy when compared with the one-size-fits-all solution—namely, 4.4 kWh and 0.6 kWh for the logistical resupply and emergency delivery missions, respectively. We see that the logistical UAV expends more energy for the same mission, although it has a slightly lighter airframe, leading to an approximately 1 percent lower life-cycle cost. A larger difference, however, is observed for the emergency delivery UAV, where per-mission energy usage has decreased approximately 45 percent. This highlights the advantage of the mission-specific platform for this application—the smaller UAV expends less energy and is thus potentially more cost-effective, given the shorter mission.

Figure 4.4 gives the corresponding cost sensitivities. As was the case for the one-size-fits-all UAV, the logistical UAV is most sensitive to the minimum range constraint, followed by the payload size. The emergency UAV cost, however, is driven by the operating environment that sets the necessary heat transfer characteristics of the cooling system. For example, life-cycle cost is most sensitive to the assumed difference between the ambient temperature and the blood storage temperature as well as the assumed storage time. A 10-percent increase in either, which leads to an increase in payload weight, would yield an approximate 4-percent increase in program cost. Interestingly, the emergency UAV cost is less sensitive to the number of blood units in the payload. Finally, for the logistical UAV, we observe a similar sensitivity to response time as was seen for the one-size-fits all solution (i.e., an approximately 0.1-percent increase in cost for a 10-percent decrease in response time). However, the cost of the emergency delivery vehicle is an order of magnitude more sensitive to its corresponding response time (i.e., a 10-percent decrease yields an expected 1-percent increase in cost).

We draw two conclusions from this analysis. First, the logistical resupply mission drives the design of the one-size-fits-all UAV, given the similarity between it and the corresponding mission-specific plat-

Figure 4.4
Cost Sensitivities (Percent Change in Life-Cycle Cost for a 1-Percent Change in Mission Parameter) for the Two Mission-Specific UAVs

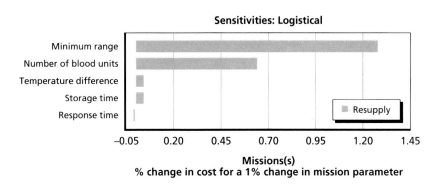

SOURCE: RUDOFF tool.

form. Second, life-cycle costs of the two mission-specific platforms are most sensitive to different mission parameters. Range constraints drive the design of the logistical resupply aircraft while payload requirements drive the cost of the emergency delivery UAV. The latter platform, however, is not insensitive to the minimum mission range. This result illustrates that acquiring additional capability for different mission sets has different cost implications. RUDOFF allows program analysts to understand and visualize these potential trade-offs.

Using RUDOFF to Select the Optimal Platform-Mission Assignment

Previously, we assumed that the "optimal" assignment of missions to platforms was one-to-one. In general, however, this is not necessarily the case. For example, the "optimal" choice could be the one-size-fits-all solution. Alternatively, there is no reason why multiple platforms could not be used for the same mission space—that is, one UAV for one subset of logistical resupply missions and a second for the remaining. Ideally, we would then like a tool that can make that optimal selection for us.

Using RUDOFF's outer fleet optimization model, previously described in Chapter Three, we can estimate the optimal platform/mission combination.[9] In this case, we assume that both the inner and outer model objective functions are identical (i.e., the fleet objective function is also the total life-cycle cost of all platforms). Table 4.4 gives the resulting normalized fleet objective function values as a function of the number of platforms.[10] In the two examples where mission-specific platforms are assumed, we consider two separate cases: (1) The mission space requires a total of 10 aircraft—eight for logistical missions and two for emergency missions, and (2) the mission space requires a total of 12 aircraft—eight for logistical missions and four for emer-

Table 4.4
RUDOFF Fleet Objective Function Results for the Mission Assignment Example

Number of Platforms	Number of Units	Normalized FOF
1	10	1.25
2	8/2	1.01
2	8/4	1.00

SOURCE: RUDOFF tool.

NOTE: For the two-platform cases, the "Number of Units" column corresponds to the number of logistical resupply/emergency delivery UAVs, respectively.

---

[9] Note that because the mission assignment problem is solved using a heuristic approach, global or local optimality cannot be guaranteed. Future model improvements will focus on refining solution methods.

[10] Because we have only defined two missions in the mission space, the mission assignment problem assuming three UAV platforms is not well posed; thus, we only compare the one-size-fits-all and mission-specific examples.

gency missions. The second case is meant to represent the fact that using a fleet with mission-specific platforms will likely create substitution issues. Whereas in the one-size-fits-all case, that UAV could fly either mission, demand could be further constrained if the mission-appropriate platform is not currently on-station, even if the same total number of platforms is the same. In other words, 10 mission-specific platforms are not necessarily equivalent to 10 one-size-fits-all UAVs when attempting to meet total mission demand. A more detailed assessment of substitutability and its impact on fleet composition is currently outside the scope of this analysis, but future analyses could incorporate expected mission demands when sizing fleets of mission-specific or multi-mission UAV platforms.

As these results show, RUDOFF estimates the optimal mission assignment to be the one-size-fits-all platform (larger normalized FOFs are better), because the additional cost to develop and procure two mission-specific platforms outweigh the mission-specific advantages. Note that different definitions of the fleet objective function (i.e., including other sustainment costs) can certainly change the outcome. In this case, mission energy costs are small compared with the development and unit costs, biasing the fleet optimization solution toward a fewer number of platforms, even though there are clear inefficiencies associated with flying a larger aircraft in the emergency delivery role.

Finally, we note that the mission assignment example explored in this analysis is trivial—there exists only one possible assignment for each case. Future analyses can use RUDOFF to assess a larger set of possible missions, where the assignment problem becomes more complex, yielding insights that are potentially less intuitive. Also, as mentioned in Chapter Three, the FOF we used in this example did not consider redundancy in mission assignments to platforms. Future discussions with the Joint medical community should focus on which medical resupply missions should be redundant across platforms to ensure sufficient risk mitigation.

CHAPTER FIVE

Conclusions and Future Work

This analysis has assessed the utility of small UAVs for blood delivery missions. We began by describing the use of autonomous UAVs, noting their growing popularity, increasing availability, and the high level of interest in their use from the Joint medical community. We then surveyed relevant topics pertaining to the use of small UAVs for delivering blood. These topics included whether transport on small UAVs significantly degrades blood quality, the benefits of using air vehicles for alleviating logistical strain in the blood supply network, and the improvement in survival outcomes associated with starting blood transfusions as soon as possible after traumatic injury. Based on this topic survey, we presented a notional blood delivery mission space consisting of two missions: (1) logistical resupply of 10 blood units over a distance of approximately 100 miles and (2) emergency delivery of two blood units within 15 miles of an MTF.

We then described the design optimization tool, RUDOFF, developed to inform issues of importance and relevance to medical community and UAV program stakeholders. These issues include how large a blood delivery platform should be, the approximate life-cycle cost of a cost-minimized design, and how sensitive that cost is to the mission space parameters. We performed a case study using RUDOFF to optimize the design of a blood delivery UAV that flies both logistical resupply and emergency delivery missions and found that the one-size-fits-all solution's life-cycle cost (which in this case includes estimates of platform development, unit procurement, and mission energy costs) is most sensitive to the minimum delivery range of the logistical resupply mission.

We also performed several sensitivity studies, including an energy-efficiency and cost comparison between the baseline battery-powered UAV and a gas-powered aircraft that flies the same missions. While the overall efficiency (i.e., the useful power supplied to the aircraft divided the power pulled from the battery) of the electric UAV is higher, the gas-powered platform is lighter, which implies a lower unit cost. We also assessed the benefit of mission-specific UAV platforms (i.e., a flight vehicle designed specifically for each of the two mission types). Our findings are that the one-size-fits-all UAV is similar in design to the logistical resupply UAV and that the emergency UAV is more efficient than the one-size-fits-all for the emergency delivery mission, a result that follows from aircraft performance first principles. The one-size-fits-all UAV is larger and heavier than the emergency UAV and thus requires more energy to fly the same distance and carry the same payload. We also found that the logistical UAV is sensitive to the same mission parameters as the one-size-fits-all solution, given the similarity of the vehicles, whereas the life-cycle cost of the emergency delivery platform is most sensitive to the heat transfer parameters that in part set the weight of the payload.

RUDOFF also has the ability to select optimal assignment of missions to UAV platforms that minimizes a fleet objective function. We concluded this analysis by presenting a simple fleet design example, based on the previously defined life-cycle cost objective function, and using it as our fleet objective function, we estimate the optimal number of unique platforms in the blood delivery fleet. We found the one-size-fits-all solution to be the better (i.e., lowest cost) option, even though an emergency-specific UAV would achieve lower mission energy costs. We note, however, that different fleet objective functions may yield different results; therefore, care should be taken to define FOFs that accurately reflect stakeholder priorities.

Finally, there are certainly limitations to our analysis given the simplifying assumptions made throughout. Most notably, we recognize that fleet sustainment costs have a variety of components, both in terms of labor and replacements parts, that are not treated explicitly in this study. We also did not consider issues related to mission redundancy across platforms within a UAV fleet, a requirement that could be specified within a given fleet objective function. This analysis, while focused on blood delivery, is also relatively narrow in scope because it considers one concept of operations in our selected two mission spaces. Additional sensitivity studies could, for example, consider more extreme temperature conditions (e.g., both very hot and very cold environments), more heavily loaded vehicles (e.g., additional delivered units), or faster deliveries (e.g., lower emergency delivery thresholds than the 15-minute delivery time used here). Continuing engagements with the Joint medical community will help to improve and validate blood delivery mission sets to maximize medical utility.

Improving RUDOFF

RUDOFF should be considered a conceptual design tool most useful for initial trade space analyses. As discussed in Chapter Three, GP formulations are also inherently restrictive, and certain levels of fidelity may simply not be possible. That being said, there are several ways in which future users and developers of RUDOFF can improve it. First, different payload models that reflect other mission types can be readily added, given the model's object-oriented structure. Second, some of the underlying physics models should be revisited, in particular the structural and weight models, which we tuned to be most applicable to small UAV design problems. Improving the built-in physics could make RUDOFF generalizable to other design problems (e.g., optimizing Class 3–5 UAVs).

Finally, the outer model that performs the fleet design optimization currently struggles with high-dimensional problem spaces, such as a large number of missions in the mission set. To make these large problems more computationally tractable, development should focus on taking advantage of any underlying objective function structure to make use of faster combinatorial optimization solution methods. If such structure does not exist, future developers should consider alternative formulations of the mission assignment problem or other heuristic approaches.

Integrating RUDOFF with Existing RAND Tools

RUDOFF is only one of many design optimization tools, including RAND's ACES, and researchers should understand that it is most appropriately applied in the conceptual design phase and initial scoping exercises, such as the analysis performed here. As highlighted in this report, we believe this tool is most useful to stakeholders at the beginning of potential acquisition programs to understand high-level trends (e.g., as minimum mission range increases by X percent, cost increases by Y percent) and to obtain these trends very quickly. If researchers require higher-fidelity results—for example, more accurate aerodynamic performance, weight estimates, or aircraft form factors—then they are best served using more detailed (but likely more computationally expensive) models. That does not, however, rule out the use of RUDOFF in these higher-fidelity studies. For example, RUDOFF could be used to generate designs that downstream modelers use to initialize solutions for more complex models.

Future Applications

We consider this analysis an initial assessment of a single medical resupply application that sits within a much larger mission space. A logical extension of this work is to perform similar assessments of other medical resupply missions, including developing a single platform that serves a variety of purposes beyond the two assumed in this analysis. RUDOFF can also be more broadly used for other mission types (e.g., intelligence gathering, reconnaissance, other logistical support), and stakeholders and researchers can generate similar information for any application as presented in this report. Assessments of multipurpose UAVs are also possible, such that the mission space could include both reconnaissance and delivery missions. Finally, although we did not include this capability in the current version of the model, it would also be useful to compare optimized designs with existing UAV platforms to determine if new acquisition programs are even necessary.

RUDOFF Model Description

This appendix gives more technical details of RUDOFF, including descriptions of the *Aircraft* and *Mission Flier* objects as well as the implementation of the fleet optimization (outer) model. A more complete and detailed technical manual is planned for the future.

Aircraft Object

The *Aircraft* object contains all of the relevant information regarding the physical UAV, including its dimensions, geometry, and weight. The two primary sub-objects are the *Airframe* and *Power System*.

Airframe

The *Airframe* captures the dimensions of each of the primary components of the UAV. In this case, these components are the wing, fuselage, and empennage. The empennage is further composed of the vertical and horizontal tails. The wing is defined by its airfoil thickness, span, and taper ratio. The thickness is in part set by the necessary aerodynamic performance of the UAV as well as the structural constraints. The fuselage is assumed to be rectangular, with a corresponding width, height, and length. The fuselage also has a skin-thickness variable that is set according to the bending moment induced by the weight of the aircraft. The user sets the geometry of the horizontal (h) and vertical (v) tails using typical values of the corresponding tail volume coefficients, which are defined as

$$V_h = \frac{S_h l_h}{Sc}$$

$$V_v = \frac{S_v l_v}{Sb},$$

respectively, where S is the platform area of the corresponding component (no subscript denotes the wing), c is the average wing chord, l is the corresponding moment arm for each tail surface, and b is the wingspan. Typical values for V_h and V_v are 0.45 and 0.035, respectively (Drela, 2014).

Total weight of the airframe is estimated by summing the estimated weight of each of the components as follows:

$$W_{airframe} = W_{wing} + W_{empennage} + W_{fuselage}.$$

The weight of the wing is estimated using a bottom-up approach by calculating the weight of the wing spar and skin. The latter is scaled using estimated skin weights from comparably sized small UAVs. The weight of the horizontal and vertical tails is scaled from the wing by planform area. Finally, the fuselage weight is partly specified by the user and also estimated based on the computed fuselage bending moment with a scaling factor.

Power System

The *Power System* is composed of the energy source (hydrocarbon fuel or battery), the engine or electric motor, and the propeller. Engine weight is estimated using the same empirical relation to maximum required power as in Hoburg and Abbeel (2014), although other relationships are possible.[1] Propeller performance is derived from actuator disk theory, presented as

$$\eta_p = \frac{2}{1 + \left(\dfrac{2T}{Au_0 \rho} + 1 \right)^{0.5}},$$

---

[1]   See, for example, Raymer (1999).

where T is the thrust generated by the propeller, u_0 is the flight speed of the UAV, A is the propeller area, ρ is the density of the surrounding atmosphere, and η_p is the propulsive efficiency of the propeller. As in Hoburg and Abbeel (2014), a viscous penalty is applied to this ideal propeller efficiency. The total power system is then sized based on the required power for flight. The weight of the power system is similarly estimated from the weights of its components as follows:

$$W_{PS} = W_{engine} + W_{ES} .$$

Mission Flier Object

The *Mission Flier* object interacts with the Aircraft object to fly the missions defined by the user. Its primary components include the Mission model, which tracks the vehicle state along each defined leg of the mission; and a set of performance models to capture the aerodynamic, structural, and overall flight performance of the vehicle. Each is discussed in greater detail in the following sections.

Mission Model

The *Mission* model tracks the state of the UAV as it traverses each leg of each user-defined mission in the mission space. This model imposes mission constraints: minimum/maximum cruise velocity, minimum/maximum operating altitudes, minimum endurance, and minimum range. For the blood delivery case, this model also imposes the necessary response and blood storage times. In addition, it tracks the vehicle state defined by its velocity and overall efficiency and applies the fundamental flight equations for steady-level flight (i.e., thrust = drag and lift = weight). Finally, it creates all related performance objects that ultimately determine the design and necessary performance of the vehicle—namely, the aerodynamic, structural, flight performance, and engine models. Each of these performance models is described in more detail in the next section.

Performance Models
Aerodynamic Performance Model

The aerodynamic performance model is similar to that of Hoburg and Abbeel (2014), although we expand it to ensure it captures small UAV flight regimes (i.e., low Reynolds number flight). Profile drag of the wing and tail surfaces are estimated from GP-compatible regressions of XFOIL[2] outputs that give drag coefficient as a function of span-averaged Reynolds number (Re), lift coefficient, airfoil thickness, and user-specified National Advisory Committee for Aeronautics (NACA) airfoil family. Note that wing sweep is not currently implemented in RUDOFF. Induced drag is estimated using lifting-line theory using the formula

$$C_{D,i} = \frac{C_L^2}{e\pi A},$$

where $C_{D,i}$ is the induced drag coefficient, A is the wing aspect ratio, and e is the span efficiency factor. e can be formulated as a function of A and the wing taper ratio, which we account for using a GP-compatible regression derived from Drela (2014). We estimate drag on the horizontal and vertical tail using similar regressions of XFOIL data, where NACA 0010 airfoils are assumed for both surfaces. Tail configuration drag penalties are also applied and are taken from Raymer (1999). RUDOFF currently assumes a "conventional" figuration (e.g., that of a Boeing 737). Finally, we estimate the fuselage skin friction coefficient using Prandtl's empirical relation for turbulent flow over a flat plate, or

$$C_{f,f} = \frac{7}{6} \cdot \frac{0.027}{Re_f^{\frac{1}{7}}},$$

where $C_{f,f}$ is the skin friction coefficient of the fuselage and Re_f is the fuselage Reynolds number. Multiplying $C_{f,f}$ by the fuselage cross-

---

[2] XFOIL is a two-dimensional airfoil performance model. See Drela (1989) for more details.

sectional area yields the fuselage drag coefficient, $C_{D,f}$. Total vehicle drag is then summed across all components.

Structural Performance Model

The structural performance model estimates three quantities: (1) the wing bending moment, (2) the wing shear stress, and (3) the fuselage bending moment. The model then constrains these quantities such that they do not exceed material limits with an applied safety margin. The model is currently similar to Hoburg and Abbeel (2014)—that is, the spar has a box configuration whose horizontal struts take the majority of the bending forces, and the vertical struts take the majority of shear forces. It also assumes the spar is made of aluminum, although this can be easily changed to other materials such as steel or carbon composites. The fuselage bending moment is similarly constrained to not exceed material limits, assuming the fuselage is made of a composite material.

Flight Performance Model

The flight performance model estimates fuel burn as a function of distance flown for a given mission segment. For UAVs with internal-combustion engines, the linearized Breguet Range equation as derived by Hoburg and Abbeel (2014) is applied. For the electric system, however, range and endurance are modeled as functions of battery discharge times; that is, UAV endurance is equal to the battery discharge time, and range is equal to the discharge time multiplied by the flight speed.

Engine Performance Model

The engine performance model estimates the amount of fuel burn or necessary battery weight as a function of distance flown in each mission segment. RUDOFF estimates these quantities based on the total power consumption of the UAV, which is the power delivered to the aircraft divided by the estimated overall efficiency, as follows:

$$P_{total} = \frac{Tu_0}{\eta_o} .$$

It also applies volume constraints to ensure that there is room to carry the fuel or batteries within the fuselage. Finally, it constrains the allowable propeller tip speed to be lower than the speed of sound (i.e., Mach 1), the typical performance limit for such systems. The engine model does not currently calculate optimal engine/motor operating points, where the user specifies the motor revolutions per minute (rpm). For the internal combustion case, fuel parameters are based on aviation gasoline. For the electric motor case, battery parameters are based on lithium-ion cells. The engine performance model does not currently model battery performance as a function of drawn power, as effective cell capacity decreases with increasing power requirements.

Fleet Optimization

This section briefly describes the (outer) fleet optimization model in greater detail. First, we describe how we formulated the fleet design search as a combinatorial optimization problem—more specifically, an assignment problem. Then, we describe two implemented methods to solve the corresponding problem: (1) an exhaustive search and (2) a heuristic search using a genetic algorithm. Finally, we present a validation case of the outer model.

Formulating Fleet Design as an Assignment Problem

As outlined in Chapter Three, we cast fleet design as a mission assignment problem: For a given number of unique platforms, we want to know which subset of missions should be assigned to each vehicle. The goal is to assign all missions in the user-defined mission space, but this is not necessarily feasible. Figure A.1 gives a more generalized description of the mission assignment problem than is given in

Figure A.1
Generalized Visualization of the Mission Assignment Problem

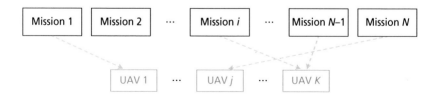

Figure 3.2. More specifically, the objective is to assign as many of the N missions to K UAVs to maximize a user-defined objective function, previously referred to as the fleet objective function, or FOF. As indicated in the Figure A.1, every UAV must have at least one mission assigned to it, otherwise there would be no reason not to consider K – 1 platforms instead. Also, not all missions need to be assigned to a UAV because that could generate infeasible designs. FOFs, however, can be defined to penalize those sets of assignments that do not span the entire mission space.

Typically, solution algorithms attempt to take advantage of some problem structure to more efficiently solve combinatorial optimization problems. Currently, RUDOFF does not exploit any problem structure using more sophisticated algorithms. Given this constraint, we have so far implemented two solution routines: (1) an exhaustive search and (2) a heuristic search using a genetic algorithm. Each approach needs to be explained in more detail.

Regarding the exhaustive search, the simplest case is assigning a given number of missions to a single platform. The optimal solution is to assign all missions to the vehicle.[3] If this is not feasible, then the algorithm considers all possible combinations of sets of N – 1 missions.[4] If RUDOFF finds no feasible set of assignments, then combinations of N – 2 missions are considered and so on. Considering multiple UAV platforms complicates the problem as the possible combinations of missions must then be divided into K subsets. This latter set of combinations is known as a Stirling number of the second kind, which quickly encounters dimensionality issues. For example, there are more than 45 billion ways to assign 20 missions to four UAVs. Regardless, the exhaustive search looks through all possible combinations to locate the optimal assignment. A way to reduce the number of combinations that RUDOFF considers is to start with the largest set of possible missions and work backward—the search ends once a feasible solution is

---

[3]   Note that this statement may not be strictly true, as it depends on how much the user values span the entire mission space versus the cost of the corresponding UAV. There could be instances where a mission could be omitted if it generates enough cost-savings.

[4]   In combinatorics parlance, this would be "N choose N – 1" combinations.

found—but this does not necessarily guarantee that the global optimum has been located.

To avoid dimensionality issues inherent to the exhaustive search, we also implement a heuristic search using a genetic algorithm. GAs use concepts from evolutionary biology to "evolve" populations toward an approximately optimal solution. Populations, in this case, refer to UAV designs. The evolutionary process includes steps to "mate" better-performing solutions and stochastically mutate designs to move toward better-performing sets of populations while also avoiding local optimums. We implement a GA search in RUDOFF using the Distributed Evolutionary Algorithms in Python (DEAP) library. The validation case in the next section uses the GA search.

Validating the Outer Fleet Optimization Model

We also conducted a validation of the outer model using a highly stratified mission space—that is, a group of short, fast missions and a group of long, slow missions—and compared results when assuming mission allocations to one, two, and three different UAV platforms. The fleet objective function for this validation follows from Equations (2) and (3) in Chapter Three. We use the weight of the UAVs as a proxy for unit cost and the energy consumption for a given UAV-mission pairing as a proxy for mission lifetime cost, and then approximate the development cost to be some fixed multiple of the unit cost. Table A.1 outlines the assumptions within the FOF for this validation case. Note that for the unit cost, we assume that 10 UAVs are required for each mission, setting the number of procured units. For operational costs, we assume

Table A.1
Assumptions Embedded Within the FOF UAV Cost Function (First Term) for the Fleet Optimization Validation Case

Unit	Development	Operational
~ UAV empty weight	= 100 × unit cost	~ Mission energy consumption
10 UAVs per mission	N/A	Missions 1–5: 100 times; Missions 6–10: 10 times

Table A.2
Parameters of 10 Randomly Generated Missions Used in
Outer Model Validation

Mission	Range (km)	Minimum Cruise Speed (m/s)	Payload (kg)
1	248	0	4
2	241	0	5
3	245	0	8
4	243	0	10.5
5	202	0	4
6	23.7	55	7.5
7	24.8	55	9
8	23.3	55	12.5
9	20.7	55	2
10	21.6	55	8

that missions 1–5 are flown 100 times over the course of the fleet life-time while missions 6–10 are flown only 10 times.

The UAV fleet is optimized over 10 randomly generated missions; Table A.2 gives the mission parameters. As stated above, the mission space is stratified into two clusters: One group contains shorter but faster missions while the second contains longer, higher-endurance missions.[5] The payloads between the two clusters are comparable. We would then expect that the optimal allocation would either be all missions assigned to a single platform or each mission strata assigned to a specific platform, while allocation to three platforms would ultimately be suboptimal.

Figure A.2 shows the results from the validation case. The top panel in the figure gives the values of the objective function assum-

---

[5] "Faster" and "slower" in this case refer to the minimum imposed cruise velocity constraint on the inbound and outbound legs, not necessarily the speed at which a given mission will be executed.

Figure A.2
Values of the Defined FOF for Mission Allocations to One, Two, and Three UAV Platforms (Top); Visualization of Mission Allocation from Outer Model Validation Case (Bottom)

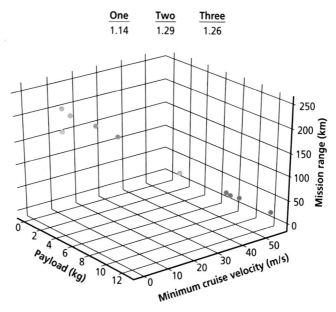

SOURCE: RUDOFF tool.
NOTE: The faster, shorter missions are assigned to UAV 1 (blue); the longer, slower missions are assigned to UAV 2 (green).

ing allocation to one, two, and three platforms, and the bottom panel shows the optimal allocation of missions to two UAV platforms. In this particular case, and as expected, the optimal solution is to assign each strata to a single UAV, implying that the FOF is structured such that the reduction of total energy cost over the lifetime of the systems outweighs the additional development cost of an additional UAV platform. Modifying the relative weights of each cost component (i.e., assuming larger development costs for a given unit cost) could shift the optimal fleet design to a single platform.

User-Defined Inputs for RUDOFF

To execute RUDOFF, the user must provide a set of inputs to properly define the optimization problem. These inputs consist of two components: (1) the mission definition file and (2) the aircraft definition file. The next sections describe each in greater detail.

Mission Definition File

The mission definition file contains the full set of missions defined within the mission space for a given analysis. Each mission is defined separately and has two corresponding categories of parameters: operational and payload. Table B.1 provides a description of these two sets of inputs.

Operational inputs define the number of mission segments and each segment's associated minimum and maximum cruise velocity and a minimum loiter time. As an example, consider a three-segment reconnaissance mission where the user imposes a minimum cruise velocity on the outbound leg, a maximum cruise velocity and minimum loiter time for the middle reconnaissance leg, and a minimum cruise velocity for the return leg. The user also specifies a minimum-range constraint that applies to each mission segment. Finally, the user must a priori set the mission altitude and associated atmospheric conditions, (i.e., density, pressure, and ambient temperature).

Payload inputs are a function of the selected payload model to be specified in the aircraft definition file. If the *simple* payload model is selected, then RUDOFF takes a user-specified payload mass. If the *blood* payload model is selected, then RUDOFF estimates the payload

Table B.1
Mission Definition File Parameters and Descriptions

Category	Parameter	Units	Description
Operational	n	—	Number of mission segments
	z	m	Mission altitude
	R_{min}	m	Minimum operating range
	V_{min}	m/s	Minimum allowable cruise velocity per flight segment. [$n \times 1$ vector]
	V_{max}	m/s	Maximum allowable cruise velocity per mission segment. [$n \times 1$ vector]
	$t_{l,min)}$	s	Minimum allowable loiter time per flight mission segment. [$n \times 1$ vector]
Payload	m_{pay}	kg	Mass of payload for *simple* payload model
	$t_{store,min}$	s	Minimum storage time of blood for *blood* payload model
	ΔT	K	Temperature difference between environment and blood cooler for *blood* payload model
	$t_{response}$	s	Delivery response time for *blood* payload model
	n_{units}	—	Number of whole blood units for *blood* payload model

mass from the corresponding heat transfer model. In addition, the minimum cruise velocity for the outbound leg is superseded by the velocity determined from the mission range divided by the required response time. Table B.2 gives the mission definition file for the emergency delivery UAV from Chapter Four.

Aircraft Definition File

The aircraft definition file specifies physical constants and some geometric specifications of the aircraft. For multiplatform analyses, each aircraft is defined separately within the file. Table B.3 provides a description of these inputs.

Table B.2
Mission Definition File for the Emergency Delivery UAV
from Chapter Four

Category	Parameter	Units	Value
Operational	n	—	2
	z	m	100
	R_{min}	m	40000
	V_{min}	m/s	[—,0.001]
	V_{max}	m/s	[1000,1000]
	$t_{l,min}$	s	0.001
Payload	m_{pay}	kg	—
	$t_{store,min}$	s	259200
	ΔT	K	15
	$t_{response}$	s	900
	n_{units}	—	2

NOTE: Because this is an example of the mission-specific
platform, only a single mission is contained in the file.

Table B.3
Aircraft Definition File Parameters and Descriptions

Category	Parameter	Units	Description
Constants	g	m/s^2	Gravitational constant
	ρ_{ES}	J/m^3	Energy source energy density
	S_{ES}	J/kg	Energy source specific energy
UAV-Engine	eng_opt	—	Engine option variable, either *electric* or *ic*
	η_{eng}	—	Engine efficiency
UAV-Wing	$C_{L,max}$	—	Wing maximum lift coefficient
	σ	N/m^2	Wing maximum shear stress
	airfoil_opt	—	Wing airfoil option variable, either *N24XX* or *N230XX*
UAV-Payload	payload_opt	—	Payload option variable, either *simple* or *blood*

The energy source parameters are either those of a hydrocarbon base fuel for the *ic* (i.e., internal combustion, engine option parameter) or a lithium-ion battery for the *electric* option. The user also defines the corresponding engine efficiency. For the wing, the user specifies a maximum lift coefficient that is set external to the aerodynamic performance model, a maximum allowable wing shear stress parameter, and a wing airfoil option, where *N24XX* and *N230XX* correspond to the NACA four- and five-digit families with variable thickness. Finally, the user also set the payload model as described in the mission definition file above. Table B.4 gives the aircraft definition file for the emergency delivery UAV from Chapter Four.

Table B.4
Aircraft Definition File for the Emergency Delivery UAV from Chapter Four

Category	Parameter	Units	Value
Constants	g	m/s^2	9.81
	ρ_{ES}	J/m^3	1750
	S_{ES}	J/kg	720000
UAV-Engine	*eng_opt*	—	*electric*
	η_{eng}	—	0.9
UAV-Wing	$C_{L,max}$	—	1.3
	σ	N/m^2	250×10^6
	airfoil_opt	—	*N24XX*
UAV-Payload	*payload_opt*	—	*blood*

NOTE: Because this is a single platform example, only one aircraft is defined.

UAV Fleet Visualization Tool User Manual

RUDOFF includes a fleet visualization tool, which we describe here in detail, including tool layout, input options, and interactive features. The tool is not currently hosted on an internal server. Please contact the authors for access.

Outline

Description: an interactive tool for fast UAV design optimization with user-defined missions and fleet assignment.

Tab 1: Missions

UAV Visualization

The tool automatically runs the algorithm with a fleet of three UAVs and a 2 kg payload for each UAV. The design of each UAV is represented using three measurements:

1. Wingspan
2. Tailspan
3. Fuselage length

Sensitivities Tornado Plot

The top sensitivities in the positive and negative direction are displayed in each tornado plot. Each plot is recalculated with each change to the payload.

Changing the Payload Weight

- Options: [1 through 20]
- Default: 2

At any time the user may change the payload weight (measured in kilograms) for a given UAV using a slider bar positioned directly above each UAV. This change will immediately trigger the algorithm to redesign that UAV and display the new wingspan, tailspan, and fuselage length.

The size of the payload is represented by the black box at the center of each UAV.

Changing the Number of UAVs in the Fleet

- Options: [1, 2, 3]
- Default: 3

The user may also determine how many UAVs are in the fleet using the slider bar at the top left. User must select from one to three UAVs. There is a known bug here; the page must be resized after changing this option because the reactive elements on the page are updated inaccurately.

Must Loiter?

- Options: ['yes', 'no']
- Default: 'yes'

This option allows the user to select if the mission requires the UAV to loiter during the mission. If user selects 'no,' a dropdown will disappear from the page.

How Long to Loiter?

- Options: [2400, 3600, 4800]
- Default: 4800

Measured in seconds. This is the amount of time required to loiter for the mission.

How Far Must You Go?

- Options: [10000 through 100000]
- Default: 4800

This is the total round-trip distance (measured in meters) the UAV must be able to travel during the mission.

Minimum Flight Velocity

- Options: [0.001 through 0.01]
- Default: 0.001

This is the minimum velocity (measured in meters per second) the UAV must be able to travel during the mission.

Maximum Flight Velocity

- Options: [65 through 100]
- Default: 70

This is the maximum velocity (measured in meters per second) the UAV must be able to travel during the mission.

Submit: Mission 1 Button
Click to submit all selected options to Mission 1 of the mission space.

Refresh Page Button
Refreshes the page.

Tab 2: Demo

The Demo tab shows the difference between the optimization output and the actual RQ-11 UAV.

Right Panel in Blue
This panel displays the actual measurements of the RQ-11 UAV's wingspan, tailspan, and fuselage length. These numbers can be compared to the values displayed in red at the bottom of the Demo tab.

Middle Panel

This is similar to the panels in the Missions tab; however, here we see two UAV visualizations, one in red and one in black:

- Red: This UAV is the one outputted by the optimization procedure.
- Black: This is the RQ-11 UAV.

Hovering over the Pareto front in the left panel will alter the dimensions of the red UAV.

Left Panel—Pareto Front

This panel is interactive. When hovering your mouse over the points on the graph,

- x-axis: fuel weight
- y-axis: aspect ratio.

Accordingly,

$$A = \frac{b^2}{S},$$

where A is the aspect ratio, b is the wingspan, and S is the wing area. Each point on the graph represents how changing the aspect ratio and the fuel weight affects the dimensions of the UAV optimization.

Bottom Panels

Each number in red represents the output of the optimization depending on the data point the user hovers over in the left panel.

Tab 3: Assignment

Left Panel—Mission Space

The mission space is represented in three dimensions represented by the payload weight, speed, and distance. Click a data point in the mission space to reveal the three panels to the right.

Right Panel

Each line graph represents one dimension of the mission space. The purpose is to view the relative size of each dimension for each point in the mission space. There is one orange point that represents the point the user selected in the mission space; the remaining points are displayed in light gray.

References

AABB—*See* American Association of Blood Banks.

AeroVironment, "Raven RQ-11A/B," data sheet, February 6, 2017a. As of February 11, 2019:
https://www.avinc.com/images/uploads/product_docs/Raven_Datasheet_2017_Web_v11.pdf

———, "UAS: RQ-11B Raven," webpage, 2017b. As of February 11, 2019:
https://www.avinc.com/uas/view/raven

American Association of Blood Banks, *Standards for Blood Banks and Transfusion Services, 31st Edition*, Bethesda, Md., 2018.

Amukele, Timothy K., James Hernandez, Christine L. H. Snozek, Ryan G. Wyatt, Matthew Douglas, Richard Amini, and Jeff Street, "Drone Transport of Chemistry and Hematology Samples over Long Distances," *American Journal of Clinical Pathology*, Vol. 148, No. 5, 2017, pp. 427–435.

Amukele, Timothy K., Lori J. Sokoll, Daniel Pepper, Dana P. Howard, and Jeff Street, "Can Unmanned Aerial Systems (Drones) Be Used for the Routine Transport of Chemistry, Hematology, and Coagulation Laboratory Specimens?," *PloS ONE*, Vol. 10, No. 7, 2015.

Antoine, Nicolas E., and Ilan M. Kroo, "Framework for Aircraft Conceptual Design and Environmental Performance Studies," *AIAA Journal*, Vol. 43, No. 10, 2005, pp. 2100–2109.

Boyd, Stephen, Seung-Jean Kim, Lieven Vandenberghe, and Arash Hassibi, "A Tutorial on Geometric Programming," *Optimization and Engineering*, Vol. 8, No. 1, 2007, p. 67.

Bryson, Mitch, and Salah Sukkarieh, "Vehicle Model Aided Inertial Navigation for a UAV Using Low-Cost Sensors," *Proceedings of the Australasian Conference on Robotics and Automation*, 2004, pp. 1–9.

Burnell, Edward, and Warren Hoburg, "GPkit Software for Geometric Programming," version 0.7.0, 2018. As of February 11, 2019:
https://github.com/convexengineering/gpkit

Business Wire, "Global Military UAV Market 2018–2028," June 29, 2018a. As of February 11, 2019:
https://www.businesswire.com/news/home/20180629005810/en/Global-Military-UAV-Market-2018-2028—-UCAVs

———, "Global Commercial Drones Market 2018–2022," August 1, 2018b. As of February 11, 2019:
https://www.businesswire.com/news/home/20180801005629/en/Global-Commercial-Drones-Market-2018-2022-Growth-Analysis

Bye, George, "Cheaper, Lighter, Quieter: The Electrification of Flight Is at Hand," *IEEE Spectrum*, August 22, 2017. As of March 4, 2019:
https://spectrum.ieee.org/aerospace/aviation/cheaper-lighter-quieter-the-electrification-of-flight-is-at-hand

Cap, Andrew P., Andrew Beckett, Avi Benov, Matthew Borgman, Jacob Chen, Jason B. Corley, Heidi Doughty, et al., "Whole Blood Transfusion," *Military Medicine*, Vol. 183, Suppl. 2, 2018, pp. 44–51.

DARPA—*See* Defense Advanced Research Projects Agency.

Defense Advanced Research Projects Agency, "Strategic Technology Office Outlines Vision for 'Mosaic Warfare,'" August 4, 2017. As of February 11, 2019:
https://www.darpa.mil/news-events/2017-08-04

Drela, Mark, "XFOIL: An Analysis and Design System for Low Reynolds Number Airfoils," in Thomas J. Mueller, ed., *Low Reynolds Number Aerodynamics: Proceedings of the Conference Notre Dame*, Berlin: Springer, 1989, pp. 1–12.

———, *Flight Vehicle Aerodynamics*, Cambridge, Mass.: MIT Press, 2014.

EIA—*See* U.S. Energy Information Administration.

Elroy Air, homepage, undated. As of June 14, 2019:
http://www.elroyair.com

Embention, "Veronte Products," webpage, undated. As of June 14, 2019:
https://products.embention.com/veronte/

FAA—*See* Federal Aviation Administration.

Federal Aviation Administration, "Fact Sheet—Small Unmanned Aircraft Regulations (Part 107)," July 23, 2018. As of February 11, 2019:
https://www.faa.gov/news/fact_sheets/news_story.cfm?newsId=22615

Hoburg, Warren, and Pieter Abbeel, "Geometric Programming for Aircraft Design Optimization," *AIAA Journal*, Vol. 52, No. 11, 2014, pp. 2414–2426.

Holcomb, John B., "Optimal Use of Blood Products in Severely Injured Trauma Patients," *ASH Education Program Book*, No. 1, 2010, pp. 465–469.

Javorsek, Dan, "CONverged Collaborative Elements for RF Task Operations (CONCERTO)," Defense Advanced Research Projects Agency, 2019. As of February 11, 2019:
https://www.darpa.mil/program/converged-collaborative-elements-for-rf-task -operations

Jones, Jimmy, "System of Systems Integration Technology and Experimentation (SoSITE)," Defense Advanced Research Projects Agency, 2019. As of February 11, 2019:
https://www.darpa.mil/program/system-of-systems-integration-technology-and -experimentation

Kucinski, William, "First Operational Use of Aurora's AACUS System," *SAE International*, May 24, 2018. As of February 13, 2019:
https://www.sae.org/news/2018/05/first-operational-use-of-aurora%E2%80%99s -aacus-system

Kuhn, Kenneth, *Small Unmanned Aerial System Certification and Traffic Management Systems*, Santa Monica, Calif.: RAND Corporation, PE-269-RC, 2017. As of February 11, 2019:
https://www.rand.org/pubs/perspectives/PE269.html

Kumar, G. Ajay, Ashok Kumar Patil, Rekha Patil, Seong Sill Park, and Young Ho Chai, "A LiDAR and IMU Integrated Indoor Navigation System for UAVs and Its Application in Real-Time Pipeline Classification," *Sensors*, Vol. 17, No. 6, 2017, p. 1268.

Lohn, Andrew J., *What's the Buzz? The City-Scale Impacts of Drone Delivery*, Santa Monica, Calif.: RAND Corporation, RR-1718-RC, 2017. As of February 11, 2019:
https://www.rand.org/pubs/research_reports/RR1718.html

Malsby, Robert F., III, Jose Quesada, Nicole Powell-Dunford, Ren Kinoshita, John Kurtz, William Gehlen, Colleen Adams, et al., "Prehospital Blood Product Transfusion by U.S. Army MEDEVAC During Combat Operations in Afghanistan: A Process Improvement Initiative," *Military Medicine*, Vol. 178, No. 7, 2013, pp. 785–791.

McGinity, Ashley C., Caroline S. Zhu, Leslie Greebon, Elly Xenakis, Elizabeth Waltman, Eric Epley, Danielle Cobb, et al., "Prehospital Low-Titer Cold-Stored Whole Blood: Philosophy for Ubiquitous Utilization of O-Positive Product for Emergency Use in Hemorrhage Due to Injury," *Journal of Trauma and Acute Care Surgery*, Vol. 84, No. 6S, 2018, pp. S115–S119.

Paschkewitz, John S., "Complex Adaptive System Composition and Design Environment (CASCADE)," Defense Advanced Research Projects Agency, 2019. As of February 11, 2019:
https://www.darpa.mil/program/complex-adaptive-system-composition-and -design-environment

Pelican BioThermal, "Golden Hour Medic Series 4," webpage, 2017. As of February 11, 2019:
https://pelicanbiothermal.com/products/golden-hour-medic-series-4

Petrova, Magdalena, and Lora Koldony, "Zipline's New Drone Can Deliver Medical Supplies at 79 mph," *CNBC*, April 3, 2018. As of February 11, 2019:
https://www.cnbc.com/2018/04/02/zipline-new-zip-2-drone-delivers-supplies-at -79-mph.html

Raymer, Daniel P., *Aircraft Design: A Conceptual Approach*, 3rd ed., Reston, Va.: American Institute of Aeronautics and Astronautics, 1999.

Shackelford, Stacy A., Deborah J. del Junco, Nicole Powell-Dunford, Edward L. Mazuchowski, Jeffrey T. Howard, Russ S. Kotwal, Jennifer Gurney, et al., "Association of Prehospital Blood Product Transfusion During Medical Evacuation of Combat Casualties in Afghanistan with Acute and 30-Day Survival," *Journal of the American Medical Association*, Vol. 318, No. 16, 2017, pp. 1581–1591.

Stewart, Jack, "Blood-Carrying, Life-Saving Drones Take Off for Tanzania," *Wired*, August 24, 2017. As of February 11, 2019:
https://www.wired.com/story/zipline-drone-delivery-tanzania/

Tao, Tony S., and R. John Hansman, "Development of an In-Flight-Deployable Micro-UAV," *54th AIAA Aerospace Sciences Meeting*, 2016.

Teledyne Brown Engineering, Inc., "Joint Medical Planning Tool Methodology Manual," version 8.1, 2015.

Thomas, Brent, Mahyar A. Amouzegar, Rachel Costello, Robert A. Guffey, Andrew Karode, Christopher Lynch, Kristin F. Lynch, Ken Munson, Chad J. R. Ohlandt, Daniel M. Romano, Ricardo Sanchez, Robert S. Tripp, and Joseph V. Vesely, *Project AIR FORCE Modeling Capabilities for Support of Combat Operations in Denied Environments*, Santa Monica, Calif.: RAND Corporation, RR-427-AF, 2015. As of September 12, 2019:
https://www.rand.org/pubs/research_reports/RR427.html

Thomas, Brent, Katherine Anania, Anthony DeCicco, and John A. Hamm, *Toward Resiliency in the Joint Blood Supply Chain*, Santa Monica, Calif.: RAND Corporation, RR-2482-DARPA, 2018. As of February 11, 2019:
https://www.rand.org/pubs/research_reports/RR2482.html

U.S. Air Force, "MQ-9 Reaper," fact sheet, February 10, 2019. As of September 12, 2019:
https://www.25af.af.mil/About-Us/Fact-Sheets/Display/Article/1692860/mq-9 -reaper/

U.S. Army, *"Eyes of the Army": U.S. Army Roadmap for Unmanned Systems 2010–2035*, Ft. Rucker, Ala.: U.S. Army UAS Center of Excellence, 2010. As of February 8, 2019:
https://www.hsdl.org/?abstract&did=705357

U.S. Energy Information Administration, "Electric Power Monthly," November 2018. As of February 11, 2019:
https://www.eia.gov/electricity/monthly/epm_table_grapher.php?t=epmt_5_6_a

Valerdi, Ricardo, "Cost Metrics for Unmanned Aerial Vehicles," *Infotech@ Aerospace*, Arlington, Va.: American Institute of Aeronautics and Astronautics, September 26–29, 2005, p. 7102.

Xu, Jia, *Design Perspectives on Delivery Drones*, Santa Monica, Calif.: RAND Corporation, RR-1718/2-RC, 2017. As of February 11, 2019:
https://www.rand.org/pubs/research_reports/RR1718z2.html

Xu, Jia, David Porter Merrell, John P. Godges, and James S. Chow, *Aerospace Concept Exploration System: Architecture and Methods for an Air Vehicle Design Tool*, Santa Monica, Calif.: RAND Corporation, WR-1122-RC, 2016. As of January 30, 2019:
https://www.rand.org/pubs/working_papers/WR1122.html

Younossi, Obaid, Michael Kennedy, and John C. Graser, *Military Airframe Costs: The Effects of Advanced Materials and Manufacturing Processes*, Santa Monica, Calif.: RAND Corporation, MR-1370-AF, 2001. As of March 24, 2019:
https://www.rand.org/pubs/monograph_reports/MR1370.html

Zielinski, Martin D., James R. Stubbs, Kathleen S. Berns, Elon Glassberg, Alan D. Murdock, Eilat Shinar, Geir Arne Sunde, et al., "Prehospital Blood Transfusion Programs: Capabilities and Lessons Learned," *Journal of Trauma and Acute Care Surgery*, Vol. 82, No. 6S, 2017, pp. S70–S78.

Zipline, "About," webpage, undated. As of June 14, 2019:
https://flyzipline.com/about/